MCQ
PATHOLOGY

MCQ
PATHOLOGY

Dr Mrinalini Sant MD

Former Head of the Department of Pathology
NSCB Medical College, Jabalpur (MP)

New Central Book Agency (P) Ltd

LONDON
HYDERABAD ERNAKULAM BHUBANESWAR
NEW DELHI KOLKATA PUNE GUWAHATI

NCBA

REGD OFFICE
8/1 Chintamoni Das Lane, Kolkata 700 009, India
email: ncbapvtltd@eth.net

OVERSEAS
NCBA (UK) Ltd, 149 Park Avenue North, Northampton, NN3 2HY, UK
email: ncbauk@yahoo.com

EXPORT
NCBA Exports Pvt. Ltd, 212 Shahpur Jat, New Delhi 110 049
email: ncbaexp@ncbapvtltd.com

BRANCHES

212 Shahpur Jat
New Delhi 110 049
email: ncbadel@ncbapvtltd.com

Shop Nos. 3 & 4, Vinayak Towers
681/B Budhwar Peth, Appa Balwant Chowk
Pune 411 002
email: ncbapune@ncbapvtltd.com

Shop No. 15, Bharati Towers, Ground Floor
Forest Park, **Bhubaneswar** 751 001
email: ncbabub@ncbapvtltd.com

House No. 3-1-315, 1st Floor
Nimboliadda, Kachiguda, **Hyderabad** 500 027
email: ncbahydb@ncbapvtltd.com

GSS Shopping Complex, 1st Floor
Opposite College Post Office, Convent Road
Ernakulam 682 035
email: ncbaernk@ncbapvtltd.com

Radhamayee Complex (Second Floor)
Opp. SBI, Panbazar, Jaswanta Road
Guwahati 781 001
email: ncbaguwahati@ncbapvtltd.com

MCQ PATHOLOGY • Dr Mrinalini Sant

First Published: June 2013

PUBLISHER AND TYPESETTER
New Central Book Agency (P) Ltd
8/1 Chintamoni Das Lane, Kolkata 700 009

PRINTER
New Central Book Agency (P) Ltd
Web-Offset Division, Dhulagarh, Sankrail, Howrah

COVER DESIGNER
Soumen Paul

GOVER PRINTER
Techno Process, Kolkata

TECHNICAL EDITOR
Dr. Mita Sen, MBBS

PROJECT TEAM
Prabir Ghosh, Prodip Baidya, Pradip Biswas, Prabhat Jas

ISBN 978 81 7381 852 3

Price: ₹ 235.00

Dedicated to my husband

Dr Sharad Krishnarao Sant
Retired Principal
Government Engineering College
Jabalpur, Madhya Pradesh

CONTENTS

CONTENTS

PREFACE

Recent reforms in medical education in India have prompted the replacement of multiple-choice questions with single best answer in general pathology, neoplasia, and systemic pathology. This is the first book of its kind and provides 1000 practice single best answers in pathology for candidates taking the postgraduate entrance examinations. Undergraduate medical students who are preparing for postgraduate entrance examination can use it as a practice tool.

This book is based on recent MCI syllabus, covering the modules of didactic teaching for Bachelor of Medicine (Pathology) students and Indian Medical Association recommendations.

All the major aspects of pathology are dealt with, and are organized in sequence in the following sections: General pathology, neoplasia and cytology, haematology, cardiovascular pathology, pulmonary pathology, renal pathology, oral and salivary gland pathology, hepatobiliary pathology, gastrointestinal pathology, endocrine pathology, breast and female reproductive pathology, male reproductive pathology, bone and joint pathology, nerve and muscle pathology, central nervous system pathology, skin pathology and ophthalmic pathology.

Detailed and comprehensive explanations—rather than just brief answers—have been provided so that candidates do not have to consult textbooks for clarification, as in case with most MCQ books.

Each question has been carefully formulated to cover given topic in pathology.

I hope my efforts would meet the expectations of the students. I would greatly welcome and appreciate suggestions, comments, criticisms from the interested students and erudite teachers to help me to improve this book.

Dr Mrinalini Sant

chapter 1

GENERAL PATHOLOGY

1. Granulomas are seen in except
   A) Tuberculosis
   B) Yersinia
   C) Mycoplasma
   D) Leprosy
2. Active hyperaemia is a result of:
   A) Dilatation of capillaries
   B) Dilatation of arterioles
   C) Venous engorgement
   D) Lymphatic obstruction
3. Increased number of normal mitosis may be seen in the following except
   A) Bone marrow cells
   B) Nails
   C) Hepatocytes
   D) Intestinal epithelium
4. Which of the following electromagnetic radiation carries maximum risk:
   A) Alpha rays
   B) Gamma rays
   C) Beta rays
   D) X-rays
5. Wegener's granulomatosis affects all of the following except:
   A) Brain
   B) Lungs
   C) Kidney
   D) All of above
6. Which of the following is a disorder of growth.
   A) Dystrophy
   B) Metaplasia
   C) Atherosclerosis
   D) Hyperplasia
7. Keloid scars are made up of:
   A) Dense collagen
   B) Loose connective tissue
   C) Granulomatous tissue
   D) Loose areolar tissue
8. Which is the guardian gene?
   A) P53 gene
   B) myc proto oncogene
   C) Erb-B
   D) Cyclin D
9. Electron microscope is invented by:
   A) Metchnikoff
   B) Paul Ehrlich
   C) Ruska
   D) Lichtenstein
10. Capillary permeability is increased by
    A) Bradykinin
    B) Adrenaline
    C) Calcium
    D) Vasopressin
11. Immunoglobulin which crosses placenta is:
    A) IgM
    B) IgG
    C) IgE
    D) IgA
12. IgG has molecular weight of
    A) 10000

B) 6000
C) 15000
D) 32000

13. Amyloid depositions occurs in:
A) Hypernephroma
B) Papillary adenocarcinoma ovary
C) Medullary carcinoma thyroid
D) Carcinoid tumour

14. Chromosomal abnormality seen in criminals is:
A) XXXX
B) X0
C) XYY
D) XY

15. Chromosomal abnormality seen in Turner's syndrome is:
A) XXY
B) XYY
C) X0
D) XXX

16. Klinefelter syndrome is characterized by except:
A) Primary infertility
B) Gynaecomastia
C) Testicular atrophy
D) X0

17. Wernicke's encephalopathy is caused by:
A) Vitamin B_{12}
B) Vitamin B_6
C) Vitamin B_1
D) Vitamin B_3

18. Which condition can gives rise to metastatic calcification?
A) Sarcoidosis
B) Renal failure
C) Pulmonary tuberculosis
D) Multiple myeloma

19. Diseases associated with HLA–B-8 include except:
A) Sjogren's syndrome
B) Multiple sclerosis
C) Myasthenia gravis
D) Grave's disease

20. Factors predisposing to thrombosis are except:
A) Thrombocytopaenia
B) Polycythaemia
C) Dehydration
D) Thrombophlebitis

21. Mallory hyaline is composed of
A) Desmin
B) Pre-keratin
C) Vimentin
D) Neurofilaments

22. Long arm of chromosome 5 is seen in
A) Crohn's disease
B) Ulcerative colitis
C) Polyposis coli
D) Pheochromocytoma

23. Zoonotic disease is:
A) Syphilis
B) Leprosy
C) Anthrax
D) Tetanus

24. Rheumatoid factor may be seen in all except:
A) Typhoid
B) Syphilis
C) Pulmonary TB
D) Infectious mononucleosis

25. The human lipoprotein containing the highest percentage of triglyceride by weight is:
A) VLDL
B) Chylomicron
C) HDL
D) LDL

26. Amyloid reacts with following stain except:
A) Congo red
B) Thioflavin T
C) Methyl violet
D) Prussian blue

27. Necrosis is a feature in the following chronic inflammation except:
A) Actinomycosis
B) Syphilis
C) Sarcoidosis
D) Tuberculosis

28. Exudation of plasma and leukocytes in acute inflammation is from the:
A) Venules
B) Capillaries
C) Arterioles
D) Both B and C

29. The following are adhesion molecule found on the endothelial cell surface receptors except:
A) Selectin
B) Cytokines
C) Vascular cell adhesion molecule
D) CD 54

30. Which of the following mediators of inflammation is derived from plasma?
A) Kinin
B) Histamine
C) Leukotriene
D) Cytokines

31. Physiological giant cells are except:
A) Syncytiotrophoblast
B) Osteoclast
C) Megakaryocyte
D) Tuton giant cell

32. Which of the following mediators derived from cells:
A) Complements
B) Cytokines
C) Kinin
D) Fibrin

33. The cell most sensitive to ischemia is
A) Myocardial fibres
B) Glial cells of brain
C) Renal tubular epithelium
D) Cortical neuron

34. Which of the following hornone affect wound healing maximally?
A) Adrenaline
B) Thyroxine
C) Cortisone
D) Parathormone

35. Choose the incorrect answer Prostacyclin PGI_2
A) Decreases vasodilatation
B) Decreases vascular tone
C) Increases vascular permeability
D) Reduces platelet adhesion

36. Which is not characteristic of Meig's syndrome?
A) Benign ovarian tumour
B) Malignant ovarian tumour
C) Ascitis
D) Pleural effusion

37. Following phagocytosis micro-organisms are killed by:
A) Lysozymes
B) Lymphokines
C) Complement system
D) IgG

38. Which of the following stain is not used to demonstrate calcium in tissues:
A) Hematoxylin
B) von-Kossa stain
C) Alzarin
D) Vital staining

39. The following are useful in the diagnosis of HIV infection
A) Polymerase chain reaction
B) P24 protein assay
C) CD4:CD8 ratio
D) All of the above

40. All are zoonotic diseases except:
A) Anthrax
B) Plague
C) Diphtheria
D) Tuberculosis

41. Increase in tissue size due to increase in cell size is:
A) Hyperplasia
B) Hypertrophy
C) Metaplasia
D) Hamartoma

42. In presence of inflammation, the following are raised?
A) Platelets
B) Ferritin
C) Ceruloplasmin
D) All of the above

43. Oxygen dependent killing mechanisms found in neutrophils include:
A) Lactoferrin
B) Histamine
C) Lysosomal proteolysis
D) Hydrogen peroxide

44. Which of the following hormone affects wound healing maximally?
A) Adrenaline
B) Cortisone
C) Thyroxine
D) Parathormone

45. True about testicular feminization are all except:
A) Short stature
B) Vagina present
C) 46 XY
D) Primary amenorrhoea

46. Dr. Karry Mulis introduced:
A) Electrophoresis
B) Polymerase chain reaction
C) Southern blot
D) ELISA

47. Following an acute inflammation following may occur:
A) Complete resolution
B) Abscess formation
C) Scar formation
D) All of the above

48. Which of following is not a sex linked recessive disorder:
A) Dyskeratosis congenital
B) Haemophilia
C) G6PD deficiency
D) Thalassaemia

49. Birbeck granules are seen in:
A) Eosinophilic granuloma
B) Letterer-Siwe disease
C) Hand-Schuller-Christian disease
D) All of the above

50. Which of the following diseases can cause hypercalcemia?
A) Hypervitaminosis D
B) Milk alkali syndrome
C) Immobilization
D) All of the above

51. Eosinophilic granules in cytoplasm of convoluted tubules in cellular degeneration are:
A) Endoplasmic reticulum
B) Mitochondria
C) Golgi apparatus
D) Nuclear remnants

52. C reactive protein is present in serum except:
A) Rheumatoid arthritis
B) Myocardial infarction
C) Viral fever
D) Pneumococcal infection

53. The following promote wound healing except:
A) Macrophages
B) Myofibroblast
C) Endothelial cells
D) Apocrine cells

54. Amino acid excreted in urine in cystinosis is:
A) Cystine
B) Ornithine
C) Arginine
D) All of the above

55. Constituents of emboli are:
A) Air
B) Amniotic fluid
C) Tumour
D) All of the above

56. Touton's giant cells are seen in except:
A) Liposarcoma
B) Chalazion
C) Erdheim Chester disease
D) Juvenile xanthogranuloma

57. The following substances increases the vascular permeability in acute inflammation are except:
A) Bradykinin
B) Prostacycline
C) Histamine
D) Angiotensin

58. Histamine is released by:
A) Mast cells

B) Lymphocytes
C) Macrophages
D) Neutrophils

59. In gonadal dysgenesis chromosome present is:
A) 45, X
B) 46, XX
C) 45, X and 46, XX
D) None

60. Vitamin, which is taken to prevents neural tube defect:
A) Thiamine
B) Folic acid
C) Pyridoxine
D) Vitamin C

61. Choose incorrect answer:
A) Trisomy 18 also known Patau's syndrome
B) Is almost universally lethal
C) Is associated with choroid plexus cyst
D) Is associated with IUGR

62. Patau's syndrome is:
A) Trisomy 21
B) Trisomy 18
C) Trisomy 13
D) None of the above

63. Metastatic calcification is seen in:
A) Kidney tubules
B) Fundal glands of stomach
C) Alveoli of lung
D) All of the above

64. Characteristics of Down's syndrome is:
A) Cataract
B) Hyperthyroidism
C) AML
D) Hypersexuality

65. Following are examples of genetic diseases except:
A) Haemophilia
B) Down's syndrome
C) Colour blindness
D) Pulmonary asbestosis

66. Which of the following is an example of sex chromosome?
A) Marfan's syndrome
B) Testicular feminization synd
C) Klinefelter syndrome
D) Down's syndrome

67. Annexin V is a marker of:
A) Necrosis
B) Apoptosis
C) Atherosclerosis
D) Inflammation

68. Special stain for melanin is:
A) Lead haematoxylin
B) Schmorl's stain
C) Pearl's stain
D) von-Kossa stain

69. Phagocytosis was discovered by
A) Ehrlich
B) Metchnikoff
C) Karl Mullis
D) Ruska

70. Stain for glycogen in tissues is:
A) Congo red
B) von-Kossa
C) Best carmine stain
D) Fite Faraco stain

71. The following cause hyperglycaemia except:
A) Acromegaly
B) Primary hyperthyroidism
C) Acute pancreatitis
D) Milk alkali syndrome

72. Examples of Primary T cell deficiency includes:
A) Ataxia telangiectasia
B) Wiscott-Aldrich syndrome
C) AIDS
D) DiGeorge syndrome

73. Which of the following gene is an apoptosis inhibitor gene?
A) P53
B) Bcl-2
C) Rb
D) cmyc

74. Splenic Gaucher's cells are positive for:
A) Lipid
B) Phospholipid

C) Acid fast stain
D) Iron

75. Kwashiorkor is characterized by except:
A) Edema
B) Fatty liver
C) Microcytic anaemia
D) Bitot's spots

76. Heart failure cells contain:
A) Lipofuchsin
B) Anthracotic pigment
C) Haemosiderin
D) Melanin

77. Commonest type of actinomycosis is:
A) Thoracic
B) Abdominal
C) Cervicofacial
D) None of the above

78. Anticentromere antibodies are most commonly associated with
A) Diffuse cutaneous systemic sclerosis
B) Mixed connective tissue disease
C) CREAST
D) Polymyositis

79. Anaphylactic reaction is mediated by?
A) IgA
B) IgM
C) IgG
D) IgE

80. Prostaglandin with vasodilatory effect include:
A) PGE 1
B) PGF 2 Alpha
C) TxA-2
D) Prostacycline

81. Haematoxylin is obtained from:
A) Sea weed
B) African grass
C) Logwood tree
D) None of the above

82. Causes of multiple infarct spleen is:
A) Amyloidosis
B) Tuberculosis
C) Sickle cell anaemia
D) Rheumatic endocarditis

83. The following conditions are observed in marasmus except:
A) Hepatomegaly
B) Muscle wasting
C) Low insulin level
D) Extreme weakness

84. Causes of massive splenomegaly (> 1000 gram) are except:
A) Thalassaemia
B) Leishmaniasis
C) Chronic myeloid leukaemia
D) Amyloidosis

85. The following are true about histoplasmosis
A) Visit to a cave inhibited by bats is a significant history
B) The patient is usually immunocompromised
C) Pneumonia is usually present
D) The "histo" test is positive in the majority of cases.

86. Choose the correct answer.
A) There are 23 pairs of autososmal character
B) The Y chromosome is larger than the X chromosome
C) The cells containing Y0 chromosome are not compatible with life
D) Barr body is only positive in people who are genotypically female

87. Wound healing by secondary intention takes place. Following statements are false except:
A) When the wound does not break apart
B) When the wound edges are brought together
C) Much more slowly than healing by first intention
D) When there is irreparable skin loss

88. In a case of keloid following statements are true except:
A) Are distinguished from hypertrophic scars by their extent
B) Extends beyond the original incisional scar
C) Are common on the deltoid regions
D) Are caused by excessive deposition of fibrin in the wound

89. Following are caused by defect in the mitochondrial DNA except:
   A) Leigh disease
   B) Myotonic dystrophy
   C) Kearn-Sayer's syndrome
   D) Laber hereditary optic neuropathy
90. Fluid with low protein content and specific gravity of less than 1.012 is called:
   A) Transudate
   B) Exudate
   C) Pus
   D) Amyloid
91. The following definitions are correct except:
   A) Hypoplasia: Failure of developing organ to reach it full size
   B) Aplasia: Failure of organization of tissue into an anatomically correct organ
   C) Dysgenesis: Failure of organization of tissue into an anatomically correct organ
   D) Metaplasia: Differentiation of a mature tissue into different immature tissue.
92. True statement about vitamin B_1 include:
   A) It is water-soluble.
   B) It deficiency is responsible for beri beri.
   C) It deficiency causes congestive cardiac failure
   D) All of the above
93. Apoptosis causes except:
   A) Activation of caspases
   B) Local inflammatory response
   C) Phagocytosis of cell fragment by local macrophages
   D) Condensation of chromatin
94. Which of the statement about granulomatous inflammation is false:
   A) It is a type IV sensitivity response.
   B) It shows dominant infiltration of tissue by plasma cells
   C) Occurs in sarcoidosis
   D) Is a feature of mycobacterial infection?
95. Which of the following is not true for hereditary haemochromatosis.
   A) Gonadal failure is seen
   B) Desferoxamine is the treatment of choice
   C) Arthropathy is seen
   D) Skin pigmentation is seen
96. Following statements are true about anaphylaxis except:
   A) Occurs 24 hours after the initial stimulus
   B) Causes eosinophilia
   C) Causes degranulation of basophils and mast cells
   D) It is produced by IgE antibodies
97. Following statement are true about Down's syndrome except:
   A) It has an incidence of 1:700
   B) It is associated with age of the mother
   C) Mosaicism accounts for 2% of all Down's syndrome
   D) It is associated with congenital glaucoma
98. Compared with intracellular fluid the extracellular fluid has:
   Choose the correct answer:
   A) A greater osmolarity
   B) A higher protein concentration
   C) A lower chloride content
   D) A lower potassium ion concentration
99. Hypertrophy: Choose correct answer:
   A) Refers to an increase in cell number in a tissue
   B) Is always pathological
   C) Of the left ventricle occurs in patients with systemic hypertension
   D) Is the principle underlying cause of benign prostatic enlargement in men
100. The presence of dilated small vessels packed with RBCs is called as:
   A) Stasis
   B) Vasodilatation
   C) Vasoconstriction
   D) Engorgement
101. Miyagawa inclusions are seen in
   A) Trachoma
   B) Donovanosis
   C) Lymphogranuloma venereum
   D) Yellow fever

102. Chronic carriers are seen in except:
   A) Measles
   B) Typhoid
   C) Hepatitis B
   D) Gonorrhoea

103. Which of the following is not a feature of apoptosis:
   A) Cell shrinkage
   B) Chromosomal breakage
   C) Chronic clumping
   D) Inflammatory reaction

104. Viral cells are specifically killed by:
   A) Cytotoxic T cells
   B) Neutrophils
   C) Complement
   D) Natural killer cells

105. Chokes are seen in:
   A) Fat embolism
   B) Air embolism
   C) Amniotic fluid embolism
   D) Thromboembolism

106. All are characteristics of acute inflammation except:
   A) Small abscess
   B) Fibrosis
   C) Resolution
   D) Loss of function

107. Following are the characteristics findings in suppuration except:
   A) Presence of lymphocytes
   B) Collection of neutrophils
   C) Accumulation of tissue fluid
   D) Autolysis by proteolytic enzymes.

108. Which vitamin deficiency is the commonest cause of craniofacial anomalies?
   A) Folic acid
   B) Pantothenic acid
   C) Ascorbic acid
   D) Retinoic acid

109. Which type of the following types of necrosis is grossly opaque and chalky white?
   A) Coagulation necrosis
   B) Liquefaction necrosis
   C) Caseous necrosis
   D) Fat necrosis

110. Which of the following is a reversible damage:
   A) Karyorrhexis
   B) Pyknosis
   C) Karyolysis
   D) Swelling of endoplasmic reticulum

111. Which of the following are most frequent site of venous thrombosis?
   A) Veins of lower extremity
   B) Pelvic veins
   C) Portal vein
   D) Hepatic vein

112. Which of the following is associated with a deficiency of third component of complement:
   A) Pyogenic infection
   B) Immune complex disease
   C) SLE
   D) Hereditary angioedema

113. Which of the following components enhances the binding of antigen antibody complex to macrophages?
   A) C_1
   B) C_3a
   C) C_3b
   D) C8

114. Secretory piece is attached to IgA:
   A) In plasma cells
   B) In epithelial cells
   C) By enzyme in mucous secretion
   D) By T cells

115. Serum cholesterol is increased in except:
   A) Hypothyroidism
   B) Hyperthyroidism
   C) Diabetes mellitus
   D) Nephrotic syndrome

116. A punched out edge is a characteristic of which type of ulcer:
   A) Tuberculosis
   B) Rodent ulcers
   C) Syphilitic ulcer
   D) Malignant ulcer

117. Sjogren's syndrome is not accompanied with:
A) Rheumatoid arthritis
B) SLE
C) Chronic active hepatitis
D) Primary biliary cirrhosis

118. Which enzyme of pancreas causes fatty necrosis?
A) Lipase and trypsin
B) Cholecystokinin and lipase
C) Trypsin and secretin
D) Lipase and secretin

119. All are characteristic of Kwashiokor except:
A) Bitot's spot
B) Fatty infiltration
C) Edema
D) Macrocytic anaemia not responding to folic acid

120. Serum amylase is increased in:
A) Acute pancreatitis
B) Perforated peptic ulcer
C) Acute appendicitis
D) Strangulated intestinal obstruction

121. Leminin is present in:
A) Plasma membrane
B) Inner mitochondrial membrane
C) Outer mitochondrial membrane
D) Basement membrane

122. Gamna Gandy bodies can be seen in the spleen in all except:
A) Amyloidosis of spleen
B) Cirrhosis with portal hypertension
C) Long standing sickle cell anaemia
D) Paroxysmal nocturnal haemoglobinuria

123. Liposomes are:
A) Monolipid layer membrane
B) Bilipid layer membrane
C) Multilipid layer membrane
D) All of the above

124. First response to injury is:
A) Vasoconstriction
B) Platelet adherence
C) Margination
D) Chemotaxis

125. Virchow's triad comprises of the following except:
A) Stasis
B) Hypercoagulability
C) Trauma
D) Abnormal vessel wall

126. Following mediators promote chemotaxis except:
A) Kalikrein
B) Complement factor C_5
C) Lymphokines
D) Serotonin

127. Dystrophic calcification is seen in all except:
A) Tubercular lymphadenitis
B) Aortic aneurysm
C) Kidney
D) Heart valves in RHD

128. All are true about type III sensitivity except:
A) Serum sickness
B) Arthus reaction
C) Anaphylaxis
D) Lupus arthritis

129. The daily requirement of folic acid during pregnancy is:
A) 50 microgram
B) 100 microgram
C) 300 microgram
D) 500 microgram

130. Madura foot is characterized by all of the following except:
A) Chronic granuloma
B) Filamentous organisms
C) Spread by lymph nodes
D) Dapsone is drug of choice

131. Earliest manifestations of rickets is:
A) Rachitic rosary
B) Pigeon chest
C) Craniotabes
D) Harrison's groove

132. Rice grain calcification is seen in:
A) Dracunculiasis
B) Cysticercosis
C) Trichinella
D) Loiasis

133. Which of the following characterizes the defect in Chediak-Higashi syndrome?
A) Phagocytosis
B) Leukocyte adhesion
C) Microbial activity
D) Respiratory burst

134. All of the following causes splenomegaly except
A) Tay-Sach's disease
B) Niemann-Pick disease
C) Von-Gierke's disease
D) Gaucher's disease

135. Commonest chromosomal anomaly is:
A) Trisomy 13
B) Trisomy 18
C) Trisomy 21
D) Fragile X chromosome

136. Which is not a macrophage?
A) Monocyte
B) Microglia
C) Kupffer cells
D) Lymphocytes

137. Examples of inherited disorder of metabolism is:
A) Duchenne's muscular disorder
B) Maple syrup urine dissease
C) Patau's syndrome
D) Down's syndrome

138. HIV affects:
A) T lymphocytes
B) B cells
C) Macrophages
D) T-helper & macrophages

139. Which one of the following belongs to MCH class II molecules.
A) HLA-A
B) HLA –B
C) HLA –C
D) D/DR locus

140. Leukotrienes are secreted by all/EXCEPT
A) Macrophages
B) Mast cells
C) Basophils
D) Platelets.

141. Examples of immediate hypersensitivity are all/except
A) Atopy
B) Arthus reaction
C) Serum sickness
D) Tuberculin reaction

142. Gaucher's disease is due to:
A) Glucocerebrosidase deficiency
B) Accumulation of gangliosidosis
C) Sphingomyelin deposition
D) Glycogen deposition

143. Russell bodies are:
A) Intracellular accumulation of immunoglobulin
B) Homogenous eosinophilic deposits
C) Seen in rhinoscleroma
D) All of the above

144. Mickulicz cells are seen in:
A) Sarcoidosis
B) Rhinoscleroma
C) Rhinosporidiosis
D) Tuberculosis

145. Heart failure cells are:
A) Lipofuchsin granules in cardiac cell
B) Pigmented alveolar macrophages
C) Pigmented cells seen in liver
D) Pigmented pancreatic acinar cells

146. Orange colour of the Benedict's quantitative test implies:
A) Sugar less than 5%
B) Sugar between 0.5 to 1%
C) Sugar between 1 to 2%
D) Sugar over 2%

147. Orange colour of urine is associated with:
A) Jaundice
B) Diabetes insipidus
C) Alkaptonuria
D) Haemoglobinuria

148. Potato nodes are characteristic feature of:
    A) Sarcoidosis
    B) Lymphoma
    C) Carcinoid
    D) Tuberculosis
149. Tuberous xanthomas in tendons are caused by:
    A) Lipoprotein lipase deficiency
    B) Apoprotein C11 deficiency
    C) Hypercholestrolaemia
    D) Multiple lipoprotein deficiency
150. Commonest worldwide cause of primary immunodeficiency is:
    A) Isolated IgA deficiency
    B) Variable immunity
    C) Combined immunodeficiency
    D) AIDS
151. Bruton X-linked gammaglobulinaemia is characterized by:
    A) Decreased T cell in circulation
    B) B-cell normal in children
    C) Mutation of gene coding kinase
    D) Manifest at birth in male child.
152. All are features of DiGeorge syndrome except:
    A) Neonatal tetany
    B) Increased susceptibility to fungal infection
    C) Absence of B & T cells
    D) Thymic hypoplasia
153. NK cells provide immunity against:
    A) Virus
    B) Bacteria
    C) Fungus
    D) Chlamydia
154. Hypoglycaemia seen in:
    A) Acromegaly
    B) Cushing's syndrome
    C) Hypothyroidism
    D) Hypopituitarism
155. All of these are antigen presenting cells except:
    A) B-cells
    B) Fibroblast
    C) Dendritic cells
    D) Langerhan's cells
156. Y chromosome is always present in:
    A) Turner's syndrome
    B) Klinefelter syndrome
    C) Congenital adrenal hyperplasia
    D) Gonadal dysgenesis
157. Hurler syndrome occurs due to accumulation of chondroitin B and:
    A) Heparan sulphate
    B) Dermatan sulphate
    C) Keratan sulphate
    D) All of the above
158. Bronze diabetes is caused by:
    A) Diabetes and Addison's disease occurring together
    B) Addisonian's disease
    C) Iron overload
    D) None of the above
159. Healing of wounds is retarded by:
    A) Proteins
    B) Cortisol
    C) UV light
    D) Vitamin C
160. Apoptosis is a pathological process associated with:
    A) Cellular hyperplasia
    B) Cellular dysplasia
    C) Cellular death
    D) Cellular hypertrophy
161. The first step inhibited due to hypoxic injury is:
    A) Oxidative phosphorylation
    B) Glycogenesis
    C) Detachment of ribosomes from RER
    D) Cell shrinkage
162. Extensive cellulitis is known as:
    A) Phlegm
    B) Phlegmona diffusa
    C) Cellulitis majora
    D) Cellulitis prima

163. Metastatic calcification is seen in:
   A) Damaged heart valves
   B) Atheroma
   C) Caseous necrosis
   D) Hypercalcaemia
164. Which of the following is/are secreted by macrophages?
   A) Coagulation proteins V, VII, IX, plasmin
   B) Cytokines IL-1
   C) Growth factors
   D) All of the above
165. Examples of granulomatous inflammation is/are
   A) Sarcoidosis
   B) Tuberculosis
   C) Cat-scratch disease
   D) All of the above
166. Southern blot analysis is used to detect T&B cell neoplasms based on:
   A) Clonal arrangement of their receptor genes
   B) Hyperchromatic and anaplastic behaviour
   C) Absence of contact inhibition
   D) Absence of cohesiveness of tumour cells
167. Thrombosis due to hypercoagulability is seen in:
   A) Women taking oral contraceptive
   B) Severe trauma or burns
   C) Cardiac failure
   D) All of the above
168. Characteristic features of hypoxic irreversible injury is/are:
   A) Vacuolization of mitochondria
   B) Swelling of lysosomes
   C) Calcium densities
   D) All of the above
169. A glassy homogenous, increased eosinophilia with moth eaten appearance in a cell is indicative of:
   A) Reversible fatty change
   B) Reversible hypoxia
   C) Necrosis
   D) B&C
170. Which of the following predisposes to thrombogenesis?
   A) Endothelial injury
   B) Stasis of blood
   C) Turbulence
   D) All of the above
171. Milroy's disease is lymphedema, which is:
   A) Familial
   B) Follows filariasis
   C) Follows erysipelas
   D) A sequele to white leg

Answers

1. C) Graulomas are not seen in mycoplasma. Granulomatous lesions are seen in tuberculosis, yersinia, and leprosy. Yersinia pseudotuberculosis can cause tuberculosis like symptoms, including localized necrosis and granulomas in the spleen, liver and lymph nodes.

2. B) Active hyperaemia is due to dilatation of arterioles. It is due to dilatation of arterioles at the site of inflammation

3. B) Increased number of normal mitosis may be seen in bone marrow cells, hepatocytes, and intestinal epithelium except nails.

4. A) Alpha rays are 20 times more effective than beta and gamma rays as causing tissue damage. Alpha particle is made up of two protons and two neutrons. When alpha particles are inhaled or swallowed, however, they are especially damaging because they transfer relatively large amount of ionizing energy to living cells.

5. D) Wegener's granulomatosis is a form of vasculitis that affects lungs. kidneys, ears, trachea, skin, nervous system, heart, gastrointestinal system and brain.

6. B) Differentiation of one mature type of tissue into another type of tissue is called metaplasia. The transformation is an alteration from a less specialized cell type to more specialized cell type e.g., cuboidal epithelium to columnar epithelium, columnar to stratified squamous epithelium, fibrous connective tissue to bone, and cartilage to bone. Metaplasia is fully reversible. It may be converted into neoplasia if persists for long duration.

7. A) A Keloid is a type of scar, which depending on its maturity, is composed mainly type III or type I collagen. It is as a result of an over growth type III collagen at the site of a healed skin injury which is then replaced by collagen type I.

8. A) P53 is also known as "guardian gene".

9. C) Ruska invented electron microscope. Metchnikoff discovered phagocytosis. Paul-Ehrlich was a German scientist in the fields of haematology, immunology, and chemotherapy and Noble laureate. He is noted for curing syphilis, and his research in autoimmunity. He coined the term chemotherapy.

10. A) Bradykinin is a vasoactive protein, which is able to induce vasodilatation and hypotension, prolonged increase in vascular permeability, cause smooth muscle contraction and induce pain at the site of injection.

11. B) IgG can cross-placental barrier.

12. C) IgG has molecular weight of 15000.

13. C) Medullary carcinoma of thyroid originates from the parafollicular cells (C cells) of the thyroid. In medullary carcinoma of thyroid cellular amyloid deposits derived from altered calcitonin molecules are present in the stroma in many cases.

14. C) XYY- males inherit an extra Y chromosome their genotype is XYY. As adults these " Super-males" are usually tall (above 6 feet) and generally appear and act normal. Early studies of XYY syndrome done in European prisoner initially lead to erroneous conclusion that these men were genetically predisposed to antisocial, aggressive behavior, below average intelligence, and homosexuality.

15. C) X0 abnormality of chromosome is seen in Turner's syndrome. This syndrome is found in human females. Some of the manifestations of Turner syndrome are congenital or infantile carpopedal lymphedema, cystic hygroma in the neck, and webbing of neck skins. Skin often shows multiple pigmented naevi. Other manifestations are webbing of fingers, dwarfism, primary amenorrhoea, sterility, preductal coarctation of the aorta, Patients present with broad chest, widely spaced nipples, cubitus vulgaris, low set ears, subnormal intelligence, and red green colour blindness. Turner syndrome is at a greater risk for chronic autoimmune thyroiditis and goiter.

16. D) Klinefelter syndrome is characterized by infertility, testicular atrophy, gynaecomastia and XXY chromosomal abnormality.

17. C) Wernicke's encephalopathy is caused by vitamin B_1 deficiency. Alcoholics with thiamine deficiency sometimes develop Wernicke's disease, named after the German neurologist who described it in 1881. In Wernicke's encephalopathy, focal degeneration and haemorrhages have been described in the nuclei surrounding the ventricles, mamillary bodies of the hypothalamus, and dorsal medial areas of thalamus. The earliest change is capillary endothelial proliferation associated with abnormal vascular permeability. There is progressive dementia, ataxia, and ophthalmoplegia. If untreated the syndrome may progress to coma and death.

18. B) Metastatic calcification is a result of an increase in the level of ionic calcium in the plasma and occurs in normal soft tissues. Metastatic calcification most commonly occurs in chronic renal failure and takes the form of either benign nodular calcification or calciphylaxis. In chronic renal failure, decreased clearance of phosphates results in hyperphosphatemia. In nodular calcification, the calcifications occur in periarticular sites, and their size and number tends to correlate with the degree of hyperphosphataemia.

19. B) Diseases associated with HLA-B8 include Sjogren's syndrome, myasthenia gravis, insulin dependent diabetes mellitus, Grave's disease, rheumatoid vasculitis, celiac disease, and dermatitis herpetiformis.

20. A) Causes of thrombosis includes, thrombocytosis, thrombophlebitis, increased viscosity of blood (dehydration, polycythaemia), slowing of blood stream (cardiac failure) and endothelial injury.

21. B) Mallory hyaline are highly eosinophilic and thus appear pink on H&E section. The bodies themselves are made up of intermediate keratin filament protein. Mallory hyaline is also known as alcoholic hyaline, is an inclusion found in the cytoplasm of liver cells. They are classically found in liver of people suffering from alcoholic liver disease, alcoholic hepatitis, alcoholic cirrhosis, Wilson's disease, Primary biliary cirrhosis, and hepatocellular carcinoma.

22. C) Long arm of chromosome 5 deletion is seen in polyposis coli. The responsible gene (APC) has been localized to chromosome 5q 21. Genetic susceptibility (Chromosome 12, 16, 7, 3, 1) is a factor associated with ulcerative colitis.

23. C) Zoonosis is an infectious disease in animals that can be transmitted from animals to human beings. Examples are anthrax, rabies, brucellosis, mad cow disease, tularemia, West-Nile disease, and Bovine tuberculosis.

24. A) Rheumatoid factor is not seen in typhoid. It is seen in systemic lupus erythematosus, Sjogren's syndrome, chronic liver disease, sarcoidosis, interstitial pulmonary fibrosis, infectious mononucleosis, hepatitis B, tuberculosis, leprosy, syphilis, malaria, schistosomiasis, subacute bacterial endocarditis, and visceral Leishmaniasis. RA factor is of prognostic and not diagnostic of rheumatoid arthritis.

25. B) Chylomicrons are large lipoproteins particles that consist of triglycerides (85-92%), phospholipids (6-12%) cholesterol (1-3%) and proteins (1-2%).

26. D) Stains used for demonstration of amyloid include, Gentian violet, methyl violet, cresyl violet, von-Geison, congo red, and thioflavin T.

27. C) Actinomycosis is characterized by an abscess, sinus formation, and presence of sulphur granules. Type of necrosis is liquefaction necrosis. In tuberculosis and syphilis type of necrosis is caseation. In sarcoidosis there is no necrosis.

28. A) Exudation of plasma and leukocytes in acute inflammation is through venules. There is vascular dilatation and stasis and pavementing of leukocytes near the endothelial lining. Neutrophils pass through the endothelial gaps in the venules.

29. B) Adhesion molecules expressed on the endothelial cell surface are of two main types. 1. Selectin and members of the immunoglobulin gene superfamily and these include vascular cell adhesion molecule 1 (VMCA 1), intercellular cell adhesion molecule 1 (ICMA 1) or CD54 and intercellular adhesion molecule 2 (ICMA-2).

30. A) Chemical mediators derived from plasma are bradykinin, kallikrein, complement derivatives, Hageman factor VIII, and fibrin degradation products.

31. D) Physiological giant cells include, osteoclast, megakaryocytes, trophoblastic giant cells and giant cells in regenerated muscle fibres.

32. B) Chemical mediators of acute inflammation derived from tissues include vasoactive amines (histamine) 5HT, prostaglandin, leukotrienes, thromboxane-A2, Lipoxins, neutral phosphatase, cytokines, plasma activating factors, nitric oxides, and chemokines.

33. B) Since the oxygen is mainly bound to haemoglobin in red blood cells, and the brain among the organs that are most sensitive to inadequate blood supply.

34. C) Cortisone hinder the formation of granulation tissue, and their immunosuppressive effects may predispose to local infection.

35. A) Prostacycline PGI_2 is effective vasodilator. They increase vascular permeability, decrease vascular tone and reduce platelet adhesion and serves as chemoattractant for neutrophils.

36. B) Meig's syndrome is defined as the triad of benign ovarian tumour with ascitis, and pleural effusion that resolves after resection of tumour.

37. A) Following phagocytosis organisms are killed by lysozymes. Lysozyme is an enzyme that is destructive of bacteria and functions as an antiseptic, found in tears, leukocytes, and mucus. The enzyme functions by attacking peptidoglycans (found in cell wall of bacteria, especially Gram-positive bacteria). Complement and IgG act outside the cell.

38. D) The stains used to demonstrate calcium in tissues are haematoxylin, Alzarin and von-Kossa stain.

39. D) Tests used for diagnosis of AIDS include: Demonstration of P_{24} antigen are ELISA, HIV proviral DNA by PCR, Plasma HIV type1 RNA by RT-PCR. Tests for demonstration of antibodies are Western blot technique. Other tests include immunofluorescence, viral culture, and HIV viral load tests. Indirect tests include CD4 and CD8 count, CD4:CD8 ratio, and B-2 macroglobulin estimation.

40. C) Zoonosis is an infectious disease in animals that can be transmitted to people. Zoonotic diseases include anthrax, plague, bovine tuberculosis, mad cow disease, rabies, brucellosis, tularemia, and West–Nile virus disease.

41. B) Increase in tissue size due to increase in cell size is known as hypertrophy.

42. D) In acute inflammation, the number of platelets are raised. As are concentration of serum proteins, including C reactive proteins, transport proteins (ferritin and ceruloplasmin), complement proteins and proteins involved in coagulation.

43. D) Oxygen dependent mechanism: Toxic based radicals e.g., superoxide (O2, - hydroxyl OH), and singlet oxygen, is produced in all phagocytic cells. Microbial killing resulting from the action of these oxygen-based radicals may be direct or may be mediated by ferric ions. Reaction of superoxide with ferric ion results in the formation of ferrous ion, which reacts with hydrogen peroxide to form hydroxyl radicals. Hydroxyl radicals react with bacterial cell wall phospholipids, causing loss of bacterial cell membrane integrity (lipid peroxidation).

44. B) Steroids hinder the formation of granulation tissue, and their immnunosuppressive effects may predispose to local infection.

45. A) Testicular feminization is also known as complete androgen insensitivity syndrome has a female external appearance despite a 46XY karyotype and undescended testes. There may be vagina but no cervix or uterus. At puberty, female secondary sex characteristics (such as breast) develop but menstruation and fertility do not occur. Patient is of normal height.

46. B) Dr. Karry Mulis introduced polymerase chain reaction.

47. D) Fate of acute inflammation includes resolution, healing by scarring, and progression to suppurative stages of acute inflammation and progression to chronic inflammation.

48. D) Sex linked recessive diseases include haemophilia A and B, G6PD deficiency, Duchenne muscular atrophy, X-link agammaglobulinaemia, Febry's disease, Testicular feminization, Fragile X chromosome, and Wiscott-Aldrich's syndrome.

49. D) Birbeck's granules are rod shaped or tennis racket cytoplasmic organelles with a central linear density and a striated appearance. They are characteristic finding in eosinophilic granuloma, Letterer Siwe disease, and Hand-Schuller-Christian disease.

50. D) Causes of hypercalcaemia are hypervitaminosis D, milk alkali syndrome, and excessive mobilization of calcium from bone as in multiple myeloma, hyperparathyroidism, and hypophosphataemia.

51. B) The precipitating granules are albuminous in nature and coarsely granular substances are mitochondria.

52. C) C reactive protein is increased in connective tissue diseases, heart attack, infections, inflammatory bowel disease, lupus erythematosus, pneumococcal pneumonia, rheumatoid arthritis, rheumatic fever, tuberculosis and carcinoma.

53. D) Factors, which promote wound healing, are endothelial cells, fibroblasts and macrophages.

54. D) In cystinosis, aminoacids excreted in urine are cystine, arginine and ornithine.

55. D) Constituents of emboli are air, fat, thrombus, atheromatous material, amniotic fluid, bone marrow and malignant cells.

56. C) Tuton giant cells: These are large cells. Nuclei are usually not vesicular and are arranged in the center of cytoplasm. The arrangement resembles a ring. Tuton giant cells are seen at sites of adipose tissue breakdown and xanthoma.

57. D) Chemical mediators, which increase vasodilation of blood vessels, are histamine, prostacycline, bradykinin and nitric oxide.

58. A) A mast cell (or mastocyte) is a resident cell of several types of tissues and contains many granules rich in histamine and heparin. Although best known for their role in allergy and anaphylaxis, mast cells play an important protective role as well, being intimately involved in wound healing and defense against pathogens.

59. C) Mixed gonadal dysgenesis is a condition of unusual and asymmetrical gonadal development leading to an unassigned sex differentiation. A number of differences have been reported in the karyotype, most commonly mosaicium 45X 46 XX.

60. B) Women who take vitamin supplement containing folic acid before conception and early in pregnancy have a reduced risk of the fetus being affected by neural tube defect.

61. A) Trisomy 18 is known as Edward syndrome. Trisomy 18 (Edward syndrome) is also called "Edward's syndrome" named after the physician first described the disorder. Trisomy 18 is seen in about one in 5,000 to 10,000 live birth. The syndrome has a very low rate of survival, resulting from heart abnormalities, kidney malformation and other internal organ disorders. Some physical malformations associated with Edward's syndrome include: A small head (microcephaly), accompanied by a prominent back portion of the head (occipit), low set malformed ears, abnormally small jaw (micrognathia) cleft palate/cleft lip, upturned nose, and narrow eyelid folds.

62. C) Patau's syndrome is Trisomy 13.

Trisomy 21: Down's syndrome

Trisomy 18: Edward's syndrome

63. D) Metastatic calcification is a result of an increase in the level of ionic calcium in the plasma and occurs in normal soft tissues. Metastatic calcification principally affects the interstitial tissue of vasculature, kidney, lungs, and gastric mucosa. It can occur in various soft tissue structures, such as muscle, subcutaneous tissue, heart, peripheral vessels, thyroid, liver, spleen, and pancreas.

64. C) Cataract, hyperthyroidism and hypersexuality are not a feature of Down's syndrome. There is hypothyroidism. It is interesting to note that Down's syndrome is often associated with acute megakaryocytic leukaemia.

Other sign and symptoms of Down's syndrome are short neck, macroglossia, and protruding tongue. Patients with Down's syndrome present with intestinal stenosis, umbilical hernia, premature aging with Alzheimer's like senile degeneration.

65. D) Down's syndrome, haemophilia and colour blindness are genetic diseases. Pulmonary asbestosis is acquired disease caused by inhalation of asbestos fibres.

66. C) Klinefelter's syndrome is due to sex chromosomal abnormality XXY. Marfan's syndrome is a genetic disorder of the connective tissue. Testicular feminization is also known as complete androgen insensitivity syndrome has a female external appearance despite a 46XY karyotype and undescended testes. Down's syndrome is also known as Trisomy 21, is a condition in which extra genetic material causes delays in a way of child develops both mentally and physically.

67. B) ApoAlert Annexin V FITC, a fluorescent annexin conjugate, is highly photostable and can be used to detect apoptosis by fluorescence microscopy or flow cytometry.

68. B) Schmorl's stain uses the reducing properties of melanin to stain granules blue-black.

A modification of MacConails lead haematoxylin has been found to stain several endocrine cells producing A and D cells of the pancreatic islet, thyroid C cells, gastrointestinal enterochromaffin cells, gastric G and X cells, pituitary ACTH and MSH cells, adrenal medullary cells and chemoreceptor cells of the carotid body.

Perl's iron stain is the classic method for demonstrating iron in tissues. The section is treated with dilute hydrochloric acid to release ferric ions from binding proteins. Their ions then react with potassium ferrocyanide to produce an insoluble blue compound (Prussian blue reaction). Mercurial fixatives seem to do a better job of preserving iron in bone marrow.

von-Kossa technique for calcium is another variant of a silver stain. Calcified tissue such as mineralized osteoid is identified by the substitution of calcium with potassium and is reduced to an insoluble black silver precipitate with phosphotungstic developer. von-kossa technique is frequently used on non-calcified bone sections for histomorphometric assessment of metabolic bone disease.

69. B) Metchnikoff discovered phagocytosis.

70. C) Best carmine stain is used to demonstrate glycogen in tissues.

71. D) Causes of hyperglycaemia include diabetes mellitus, pancreatitis and carcinoma pancreas, hyperthyroidism, Cushing's syndrome, hyperaldosteronism, acromegaly, chronic liver failure, viral hepatitis and intracranial injury.

72. D) Ataxia telangiectasia disease is B and T cell deficiency disease. AIDS is secondary immunodeficiency disease not primary. Wiscott-Aldrich syndrome is B and T deficiency disease. DiGeorge syndrome is most clearly defined T cell immunodeficiency and is also known as congenital thymic aplasia / hypoplasia, or immunodeficiency with hypoparathyroidism. In those infants who survive the neonatal period, immunoglobulin production appears normal, although antibody responses are impaired, because of lack of helper T cells. Infants with these defects are extremely vulnerable to viral, fungal and protozoal infections and suffer from tetany. The immunodeficiency primarily involves cell-mediated immunity. The thymus dependent areas of lymph nodes and spleen are depleted of lymphocytes. Circulating T cells are reduced in numbers.

73. B) Bcl-2: The programmatic nature of apoptosis is well illustrated by studying lineage dependent death of cells in the nematode worm C elegans. In C elegans, genes that inhibit apoptosis have also been identified. Best known of these is CED (cell death gene) whose human analogue is Bcl_2 protein that is present in certain B cell malignancies, and that also inhibit apoptosis. The inappropriate expression of Bcl_2 described the clinical presentation of follicular lymphoma.

74. A) Gaucher's disease is called a "lipid storage disease" where abnormal amounts of lipids called "glycosphingolipids are stored in special cells called reticuloendothelial cells. Classically the nucleus is pushed off to the side and the remainder of the cell is filled with abnormal lipids.

75. C) Macrocytic or megaloblastic anaemia is present in Kwashiorkor due to folic acid deficiency.

1. It is characterized by retarded growth of the child with mental apathy, edema of feet and general symptoms of anorexia, vomiting and loose bulky stool.
2. Hair is light, dry, and brittle, with marked depigmentation or discolouration in Africa but in India there is diffuse alopecia.
3. Children with Kwashiorkor have characteristic skin lesions with alternating zones of hyperpigmentation, areas of desquamation, and hypopigmentation, giving a *'flaky paint'* appearance. Skin shows hyperkeratosis, atrophy of epidermis, parakeratosis. The lower limbs, buttocks, and perineum are usually most affected but ulcers can occur over pressure points and deep cracks in skin folds.
4. Muscles are always wasted and as a result many children may not be able to crawl.
5. The liver shows extensive fatty change with little inflammatory exudates.
6. There is atrophy of pancreas.
7. Bitot's spots are seen due to vitamin A deficiency.

76. C) In chronic venous congestion lung alveolar walls are thickened. More severe injury to blood vessels causes small hemorrhages, especially in the lung with escape of few RBCs into the alveoli. Haemoglobin of disintegrated RBCs is converted into haemosiderin, when they are taken up by macrophages, which accumulate in alveoli, known as heart failure cells.

77. C) Cervicofacial actinomycosis is the most common types of infection, comprising 50 to 70% of reported cases. Thoracic actinomycosis occurs in 15 to 20% of cases and abdominal in 10 to 20% of cases. Cervicofacial actinomycosis is a chronic infection of the head and neck occurring most often in adult males and caused by bacteria of the genus actinomyces.

78. C) Anti-centromere antibodies (ACA) occur in CREAST syndrome and occasionally in systemic scleroderma. They are rare in other rheumatic condition and healthy persons. Anti-centromere antibodies are found in approximately 60% of patients in CREAST and 15% of those with scleroderma. The specificity of this test is > 98%. Thus, a positive anti-centromere antibody finding is strongly indicative of CREAST or scleroderma.

79. D) Type I hypersensitivity (or immediate hypersensitivity) is an allergic reaction provoked by exposure to a specific type of antigen referred to as an allergen. Type I hypersensitivity reaction involve immunoglobulin E (IgE) mediated release of histamine and other mediators from cells and basophils.

80. A) Prostaglandin E1 (PGE1) has been shown to have vasodilatation and antithrombosis effects.

81. C) Haematoxylin is extracted from the wood of the logwood tree haematoxylon compechianum.

82. C) In cases of sickle cell anaemia there are multiple infarcts in spleen. Other causes of multiple infarcts in spleen include emboli from subacute bacterial endocarditis, leukaemia, and myelofibrosis. Spotted spleen with multiple small infarcts may result from polyarteritis nodosa, Wegner's granulomatosis, hypertensive arteriosclerosis, and disseminated intravascular coagulation.

83. A) Marasmus occurrence increases prior to age 1. The afflicted are often fretful, irritable, and voraciously hungry.

A child with marasmus looks emaciated. Body weight may be reduced to less than 80% of the normal weight or height.

In marasmus there is generalized wasting of muscle mass, loss of adipose tissue, stunting of growth but no edema.

There is depletion of subcutaneous fat in the arms, chest wall, shoulders, or metacarpal regions.

The skin and mucus membranes may be dry and atrophic.

Diarrhoea is frequent, many infants are hungry but some are anorexic.

Brain, skeleton and kidney are preserved, whereas liver, heart, pancreas, and digestive tract are first affected.

84. D) The causes of massive splenomegaly (> 1000 gram) are much fewer and include: Thalassaemia, visceral leishmaniasis, schistosomiasis, chronic myeloid leukaemia, lymphomas, myelofibrosis, polycythaemia vera, Gaucher's disease, sarcoidosis, autoimmune haemolytic anaemia, and malaria. Desferoxamine is not a treatment of choice.

85. A) Histoplasmosis is caused by histoplasma capsulatum. It grows in soil and material is contaminated with bird or bat dropping. It occurs in people with a reduced capacity to fight disease, for example in patients with leukaemia, and persons being treated with drugs that suppress the body's defense mechanism. Pneumonia is not always present. Patient may be asymptomatic. Positive skin test is not diagnostic of disease. Positive skin test does not mean that a person is completely immune to reinfection. A person can learn from a histoplasmin skin test whether he or she has been previously infected by H capsulatum.

86. C) There are 22 pairs of autosomes and one pair of sex chromosomes. Barr body is found in about 3% of granulocytes in female, but seldom in males (0.2%). Size of Y chromosome is same as X chromosome.

87. C) Wound healing by secondary intention heals slowly than healing by primary intention. Healing by secondary intention occurs in open wounds, because of the presence of infection, excessive trauma, or skin loss, or the wound edges come close together naturally by means of granulation tissue and contraction and are not together by sutures.

88. D) Keloids are overgrowth of scar tissue tends to overgrow in the area, sometimes producing a lump many times larger than that of the original area. Hypertrophic scar is confined to the margin of the wound. Keloids develop most often on the chest, back, and shoulder.

89. B) Mitochondrial diseases comprise those disorders that in one way or another affect the function of the mitochondria or are due to mitochondrial DNA. Examples of mitochondrial myopathies includes:

1. Diabetes mellitus and deafness.
2. Laber's hereditary optic atrophy: There is visual loss beginning in young adulthood. It is an eye disorder character-

ized by progressive loss of central vision due to degeneration of optic nerve.

3. Leigh syndrome: It is subacute sclerosing encephalopathy. After normal development the disease usually begins late in the first year of life. There is rapid decline in function occurs and is marked by seizures, altered state of consciousness, dementia, and ventilatory failure.
4. Kearn's Sayre syndrome: A multisystem variant of chronic progressive external ophthalmoplegia that also includes heart block, retinitis pigmentosa, and CNS degeneration.

90. A) Transudate is clear, watery, may be pale yellow fluid with specific gravity of less than 1.012. Protein content is less than 3 gram%. Fibrinogen content is poor and does not coagulate on standing.

91. C) Dysgenesis is defined as defective or abnormal development of an organ, especially of the gonads.

92. D) Thiamine is a water-soluble vitamin. Thiamine deficiency causes beri beri, peripheral neuropathy, Wernicke's encephalopathy, Korsakoff's syndrome and cardiac failure.

93. B) There is no inflammatory response. Other characteristics of apoptosis are: It is programmed and coordinated cell death. Physiological and pathological stimuli both cause apoptosis. There is death of single cell. There is shrinkage of cells, formation of blebs on membrane known as apoptotic bodies, and condensation of chromatin. There is phagocytosis of apoptotic bodies by macrophages. Lysosomes and other organelles are intact.

94. B) Chronic granulomatous reaction is type IV sensitivity reaction. It is caused by mycobacterial infection such as tuberculosis and leprosy, histoplasmosis, cryptococcosis, Cat-scratch disease, sarcoidosis, Crohn's disease, and aspiration pneumonia. It shows dominant infiltration by lymphocytes, neutrophils, eosinophils, and giant cells.

95. B) Haemochromatosis, the most common form of iron overload disease, is an inherited disorder that causes the body to absorb and store too much iron. Clinical features of haemochromatosis include arthritis, enlarged liver, cirrhosis, heart abnormality, impotence, early menopause, and abnormal pigmentation of skin, thyroid deficiency, and damage to adrenal glands. Phlebotomy is the choice of treatment.

96. A) In cases of anaphylaxis symptoms usually begins 5-30 minutes after ingestion. Anaphylaxis is a severe allergic reaction that is rapid in onset and may cause death. There are prominent dermal and systemic signs and symptoms. Full-blown symptoms include urticaria, angioedema, with hypotension and bronchospasm. In the classic form, mediator release occurs when the antigen (allergen) binds to antispecific immunoglobulin E (IgE) attached to previously sensitized basophils and mast cells. When mast cells degranulate whether by IgE or non-IgE mediated mechanisms performed histamine and newly generated leukotrienes, prostaglandins and platelet activating factor (PAF) are released. There is marked eosinophilia.

97. D) Down's syndrome is not associated with congenital glaucoma. Mosaicism: Trisomy 21 is usually caused by non-disjunction in the gametes prior to conception, and all the cells in the body are affected. However, when some of the cells in the body are normal and other cells have trisomy 21, it is called mosaic Down's syndrome. Mosaicism is the cause of 1-2% of the observed Down's syndrome. The incidence of Down's syndrome is estimated at one per 700 births. 80% of children with Down's syndrome are born to women above the age of 35.

98. D) The extracellular fluid has low osmolarity. Protein content in extracellular fluid is low (9 millimolar) whereas in intracellular fluid protein content is high (138 millimolar). Extracellular fluid differs from intracellular fluid (fluid inside cells) in that it generally has a high concentration of sodium and low concentration of potassium while intracellular fluid is high in potassium and low in sodium.

99. C) Hypertrophy is defined as an increase in size of cell in a tissue. It may be physiological and pathological. Hypertrophy of left ventricle occurs in patients with systemic hypertension. Benign prostatic enlargement is due to hyperplasia of acini.

100. A) Stasis is defined as dilatation of small blood vessels and packed with RBCs.

101. C) Miyagawa inclusions are seen in lymphogranuloma venereum. Halberstaedter-Prowazek bodies are seen in trachoma. Donovan bodies are present in lymphogranuloma inguinale and Torre bodies and Councilman bodies are seen in yellow fever.

102. A) Chronic carrier is a person who harbors and transmits an infectious agent for an indefinite period. Diseases with chronic carrier include hepatitis B and C infection, trichomoniasis, giardiasis, amoebiasis, Chagas disease, gonorrhoea, typhoid, chlamydia, genital herpes, syphilis, human papilloma virus, and molluscum contagiosum.

103. D) Characteristics of apoptosis are as follows:

1. Programmed and coordinated cell death
2. No inflammatory reaction
3. Cell shrinkage
4. Cytoplasmic blebs on membrane – apoptotic bodies
5. Chromatin condensation
6. Phagocytosis of apoptotic bodies by macrophages
7. DNA breakdown is internucleosomal.

104. D) Natural killer (NK) cells: NK cells are somewhat larger than small lymphocytes It comprises 10% to 15% of peripheral blood lymphocytes. NK cells are large and possess azurophilic granules and are therefore called large granular lymphocytes. They are cytotoxic but not T cells. They can kill cancer cells and virus.

105. B) Chokes are seen in air embolism. When bubbles are present in air there is burning deep pain. Breathing aggravates pain.

106. B) There is no fibrosis in acute inflammation. Fibrosis is characteristic of chronic inflammation.

107. A) Accumulation of lymphocytes is feature of chronic inflammation. Characteristics of acute inflammation are:

1. Liquefaction necrosis
2. Collection of neutrophils
3. Accumulation of tissue fluid
4. Autolysis by proteolytic enzymes.

108. A) Deficiency of intake of folic acid during pregnancy by the mother causes a risk of baby having congenital craniofacial anomalies.

109. D) FAT NECROSIS: Fat necrosis is most commonly encountered in abdominal adipose tissue in pancreatic disease and subcutaneous tissue (trauma).

Macroscopically these are small, opaque, soft, white areas giving characteristic chalky appearance.

110. D) Karyorrhexis are features of necrosis which is a irreversible process. Swelling of endoplasmic reticulum occurs in degeneration, which is reversible.

111. A) A calf vein is the common site of deep vein thrombosis.

112. A) People with C3 deficiency are susceptible to bacterial infection. C1 is related with hereditary angioedema.

113. C) C3b, which binds covalently to glycoproteins scattered across the cell surface. Macrophages and neutrophils have receptors for C3b and can bind the C3b-coated cell or particle prepared to phagocytosis. This effect qualifies C3b as an opsonin.

114. B) Subclasses IgA1 and IgA2 can exist in a dimeric form called secretory IgA (sIgA). In its secretory form, IgA is the main immunoglobulin found in mucous secretions, including tears, saliva, colostrum, and secretions from the genito-urinary tract, gastrointestinal tract, prostate, and respiratory epithelium. Epithelial cells produce secretory component.

115. B) Serum cholesterol is decreased in hyperthyroidism. Other conditions in which cholesterol is decreased are Gaucher's disease and malnutrition.

Serum choleterol is increased in:
Hereditary hypercholesterolaemia
Hypothyroidism
Diabetes mellitus
Nephrotic syndrome
Obstructive jaundice
Biliary cirrhosis
Atherosclerosis

116. C) Gummatous ulcers occur in tertiary syphilis. Most characteristic feature is punched out edge and yellowish grey gummatous tissue in the floor. These ulcers are as a result of obliterative endarteritis, necrosis, and fibrosis, and mostly seen over subcutaneous bones.

117. C) Sjogren's disease is associated with:

1. Rheumatoid arthritis
2. SLE
3. Systemic sclerosis
4. Vasculitis
5. Hashimoto's thyroiditis
6. Primary biliary cirrhosis
7. Chronic autoimmune hepatitis

118. A) Fat necrosis is most commonly encountered in abdominal adipose tissue and uncommonly in adipose tissue of the anterior mediastinum, marrow and subcutaneous tissues. In the abdomen (peripancreatic adipose tissue and omentum) it is due to pancreatic disease- most commonly trauma to the pancreas or acute pancreatitis-with the liberation of pancreatic enzymes in the surrounding tissues. The fat within the adipocytes is hydrolysed but without destruction of the cell membranes. The cell membranes of adipocytes are damaged by enzymes lipase or lecithinase and subsequently, trypsin and lipase of pancreas penetrate the cells freely; trypsin destroys the cytoplasm and lipase hydrolyses fat into glycerol and fatty acids. Glycerol is freely miscible with water and is absorbed and metabolized, while fatty acids, remaining within the cells, combined with sodium and calcium ions from the blood to form calcium soaps.

119. D) In cases of Kwashiorkor vitamin B levels are normal or elevated and megaloblastosis or macrocytic anaemia is usually attributed to folate depletion. Macrocytic anaemia responds to folic acid.

1. It is characterized by retarded growth of the child with mental apathy, edema of feet and general symptoms of anorexia, vomiting and loose bulky stool.
2. Hair is light, dry, and brittle, with marked depigmentation or discolouration in Africa but in India there is diffuse alopecia.
3. Children with kwashiorkor have characteristic skin lesions with alternating zones of hyperpigmentation, areas of desquamation, and hypopigmentation, giving a *'flaky paint'* appearance. Skin shows hyperkeratosis, atrophy of epidermis, parakeratosis. The lower limbs, buttocks, and perineum are usually most affected but ulcers can occur over pressure points and deep cracks in skin folds.
4. Muscles are always wasted and as a result many children may not be able to crawl.

5. The liver shows extensive fatty change with little inflammatory exudates.
6. There is atrophy of pancreas.
7. Bitot's spots are present in eye.

120. A) Determination of serum amylase is largely used in the diagnosis of diseases of the pancreas and in the investigation of pancreatic function. Normal range is 0-93 IU. In acute pancreatitis, a transient rise in serum amylase activity occurs within 2 to 12 hours of the onset. Usually high levels of amylase (four to six fold elevation than normal) are observed during 12 to 72 hours.

Causes of increased serum amylase

1. Following acute pancreatitis
   Pseudocyst
   Pleural effusion
   Ascitis
2. Traumatic lesions of pancreas
3. Tumours of lung
4. Tumours of ovary
5. Lesions of salivary gland
   A. Obstruction in salivary duct
   B. Surgery
   C. Irradiation
   D. Tumours of salivary glands
6. Cholecystitis

121. D) Leminin is a protein found in the extracellular matrix, the sheets of protein that form the substrate of all internal organs also called the "basement membrane".

122. A) Gamna Gandy bodies are not seen in amyloidosis of spleen. They are seen in the spleen in patients with splenomegaly due to portal hypertension and sickle cell disease. They can be seen in other conditions such as acquired haemachromatosis, paroxysmal nocturnal haemoglobinuria, and angiosarcoma. Gamna Gandy bodies are small yellow-brown, brown, or rust coloured foci found in spleen. They consist of fibrous tissue with haemosiderin deposits and probably form due to scarring at sites of small perivascular haemorrhages.

123. B) Liposomes are artificially prepared vesicles made of lipid bilayer. Liposomes can be filled with drugs, and used to deliver drugs for cancer and other diseases.

124. A) First response to injury is arteriolar vasoconstriction. Arteriolar vasoconstriction of the blood vessels leading away from the site. A momentary white or pale line appears at the site of trauma due to direct response of the vascular smooth muscle to the injurious stimulus. Arteriolar constriction when present appears to be due to a direct response of the vascular smooth muscle to the injurious stimulus. The mechanism of vasoconstriction is unknown. It may well be neurogenic or possibly due to the action of chemical mediators. With mild form of injury, the blood flow may be re-established in 3 to 5 seconds. While with more severe injury the vasoconstriction may last for more than 5 seconds.

125. C) Virchow's triad was first formulated by the German physician Rudolf Virchow in 1856.

Virchow's triad presents the three broad categories of factors that are thought to contribute to thrombosis.

The triad consists of:

1. Alteration in normal blood flow (stasis)
2. Injuries to the vascular endothelium
3. Alteration in constitution of blood (hypercoagulability)

Alteration of blood flow includes turbulence, stasis, mitral stenosis, and varicose veins.

Injuries to vascular endothelium can be caused by damage to the veins arising from shear stress or hypertension.

Hypercoagulability can be a consequence of numerous possible risk factors such as hyperviscosity, deficiency of anti thrombin III, nephritic syndrome, changes after severe trauma or burn, disseminated cancer, late pregnancy and delivery, race, age, smoking and obesity.

126. D) After escape from blood, leukocytes migrate in tissue towards the site of injury by a process called chemotaxis. Chemotaxis is the force that attracts leukocytes into the inflamed tissue. Leukocytes migrate along the chemical gradient. Thus, chemotaxis is defined as the undirected migration of cells towards a chemical attractant. The chemical mediators which promote chemotaxis are:

1. Components of the complement system, particularly C_5a
2. Products of the lipoxygenase pathways, mainly leukotrienes B_4 (LT B4)
3. Cytokines particularly those of the chemokine family, e.g., interleukin-8 (IL-8). Hageman factor substrates prekallikrein and plasminogen proactivator were found to generate chemotactic activity for human mononuclear cells upon interaction with Hageman factor fragments.

127. C) Kidneys are involved in metastatic calcification.

In dystrophic calcification the level of plasma calcium is normal and deposition is due to local changes in affected tissue. This is termed dystrophic calcification.

Causes of dystrophic calcification may be divided in to two groups

I. Calcification in necrosed tissues.
II. Calcification in degenerated tissues.

I. Calcification in necrosed tissues

A. Caseous tissue: Dystrophic calcification occurs in caseous patches in tuberculosis. Calcification is most frequently seen in caseous material and may retain the permanent hallmark of previous tuberculous lesion. It is seen in primary tuberculosis of lung, lymph nodes and primary tuberculosis of intestine.
B. Fat necrosis usually around pancreas or traumatic fat necrosis of breast.
C. Old infarcts in the heart or else where some times calcify.
D. Necrotic foci in malignant tumour
E. Thrombi: A thrombus in a vein may be calcified forming phlebolith.
F. Dead parasites: Trichinella spiralis, Echinococcal cyst, cysticercus cellulosae, schistosomiasis and adult filariasis.
G. Hamartomas: In the vicinity of bones may undergo calcification.
H. Foetus: In an occasion of ruptured tubal pregnancy in which foetus survives for while, subsequent calcification converts it to a lithopodium derived from Greek words for stone and child.
I. Myositis ossificans-Haematoma formed in muscles not only calcifies but also ossifies subsequently.

Calcification in degenerated tissues

Hyaline change in fibrous tissues

1. Dystrophic calcification is common in dense connective tissues e.g. tendons. The dura matter and scarred heart valves following rheumatic endocarditis may get calcified.
2. TUMOURS
   1. BENIGN: It occurs in tumours e.g. fibroma and uterine myomas, which become atrophic and hyaline after the menopause. Calcification is seen in thyroid adenoma and colloid goiter.
   2. Malignant: Brain sand bodies (psammoma bodies) of some meningiomas consist of concentrically arranged cells, which undergoes hyaline change followed by calcification. They are also seen in papillary serous cystadenoma of ovary. Calcified foci may be present in carcinoma breast.
3. Atheromatous Plaque: Calcification is also seen in atheromatous plaques in aorta and coronary arteries. Dead ganglion cells of the brain may show similar calcification.

128. C) Anaphylaxis is type I hypersensitivity reaction. Type III hypersensitivity reaction: It is also known as immune complex or toxic complex mediated hypersensitivity reaction. The reaction may be general (e.g. serum sickness) or may involve individual organs including skin (e.g., systemic lupus erythematosus, Arthus reaction), kidneys (e.g. lupus nephritis), lung (e.g.. aspergillosis), blood vessels (polyarteritis), joints (e.g., rheumatoid arthritis) or other organs. This reaction may be the pathogenic mechanism of diseases caused by many microorganisms.

129. C) Folic acid is the common name of pteroylmonoglutamic acid consisted of pteridine and aminobenzoic acid coupled to glutamic acid.

The main dietary sources are green vegetables (spinach), fruits as well as liver, milk, and yeast. Maximum daily requirement is normally 50 ug, which is increased to several fold during enhanced metabolic demands e.g., pregnancy, infancy and lactation.

Daily requirement of folic acid during pregnancy is 300 microgram.

130. C) Haematogenous or lymphatic spread is unknown.

MYCETOMA

Synonyms: Madura mycosis, Madura foot, Actinomycetes

Mycetoma was first reported by Gill 1842 from Madurai South India. It is therefore commonly known, as Madura mycosis or Madura foot.

Geographical distribution: The disease is prevalent in tropical and subtropical regions of Asia, Africa, Central America, Sudan, Mexico, and Somalia.

Causative agents: Mycetoma is a subcutaneous infection caused by fungi actinomycotic or maduramycotic. The common organisms are Actinomyces israelii or Nocardia, Asteroides and Streptomyces madurae or Madurella mycetomatis.

Sites: The infection results in a granulomatous, inflammatory response in the deep dermis and subcutaneous tissue, which can extend to the underlying bone. The body parts affected most commonly are the foot or lower legs, with infection of the dorsal aspect of the forefoot being typical. The hand is the next most common location, however anywhere on the body.

Clinically: Initially subcutaneous swelling is present, followed by subcutaneous nodule. Eventually, massive swelling with induration, rupture of the skin, and formation of sinus tracts occurs. The fungal grain discharge from sinuses is thin and serous and contains the diagnostic "golden yellow" granules called **sulphur granules.** The material discharged from the sinuses is in the form of grains consisting of colonies of fungi or bacteria. They are 1 to 3 mm in diameter but may coalesce and form larger aggregations, several millimeters in diameter.

Histologically: The granule is found to contain entangled mycelia in the center embedded in pus, forming minute abscesses with a large number of monocytes, polymorphs and plasma cells. The diagnostic feature is the presence of granules

131. C) 1. Skeletal deformities in rickets:

(a) The earlier bony lesions are often cranio tabes—small rounded unossified area in the membranous bones of skull.

(b) Bony pain and tenderness over arms, legs, spine, and pelvis.

(c) There are presences of bony bumps on the ribs called *rachitic rosary* (bead like prominences) at the junction of ribs with their cartilages.

(d) Later features are bossing of the frontal and parietal bones and delayed closure of the anterior fontanelle.

(e) Extremities: Knock-knees, bow legs, and coxa vara. The bones are soft due to non-deposition of calcium salts and hence they are easily bent by the weight of the body.

(f) Forward projection of breast-bone (*pigeon chest*).

(g) Spine deformities: Spine curve abnormalities including scoliosis and kyphosis.

Harrison's grooves: The inward pull at the margins of diaphragm creates Harrison's grooves, girdling the thoracic cavity at the lower margin of the rib cage.

132. B) Rice grain calcification is characteristic of Cysticercosis. The calcified cysticercus produces (single) or multiple (often several hundred) calcifications in the soft tissues, which are linear or oval in shape and usually measure 4-10 mm or more in length and 2.5 mm in width.

The classic findings are multiple elongated foci of calcification just about the shape and size of grains of rice. These "rice grain" calcifications are usually oriented along the direction of muscle fibres. It may also occur in brain.

Dystrophic soft tissue calcification is seen in:

1. Cysticercosis
2. Dracunculiasis
3. Trichinella
4. Loiasis
5. Onchocerciasis

133. A) Chediak-Higashi syndrome, a rare inherited childhood disease characterized by the inability of white blood cells called phagocytes to destroy invading microorganism. Normally phagocytes eliminate microorganism through a process called phagocytosis, a type of cellular eating in which the phagocyte engulfs and digests a microbe by means of chemicals contained in vesicles. In individuals the Chediak-Higashi syndrome, the phagocytes have large, abnormally formed vesicles that make the cells more rigid, less mobile, and unable to destroy microorganims.

134. C) There is no splenomegaly in cases of von-Gierke's disease.

Causes of splenomegaly

Due to disturbances of lipoid metabolism

Amyloidosis, Gaucher disease, Niemann-Pick

Hand Schuller Christian- syndrome

Mucopolysaccharidoses, Letterer-Siwe disease

Tay-Sach's disease

135. C) Commonest chromosomal abnormality is trisomy 21 (Down syndrome). Trisomy 13 and 18 are more severe than Down syndrome, but unfortunately less common.

136. D) Lymphocytes are not macrophages.

A majority of macrophages stationed at strategic points where, microbial invasion or accumulation of dust is likely to occur.

Each type of macrophage, determined by its location, has a specific name:

Table showing name of macrophage and location of cell

Name of cell	Location
Neutrophils	Blood, bone marrow
Monocyte	Blood
Dust cells/macrophages	Pulmonary alveolus of lungs
Histiocytes	Connective tissue
Kupffer cells	Liver
Microglia	Neural tissue
Epitheloid cells	Granulomas
Osteoclast	Bone
Sinusoidal lining cells	Spleen
Intraglomerular mesangial cells	Kidney
Giant cells	Connective tissue

137. B) Maple syrup urine disease (MSUD), also called branched-chain ketoaciduria, is an autosomal recessive metabolic disorder affecting branched-chain amino-acids. It is one type of organic aciduria.

An infant characterizes the disease by the presence of sweet-smelling urine, with an odour similar to maple syrup. Infants with this disease seem healthy at birth but if left untreated suffer severe brain damage and eventually die.

From early infancy symptoms of the condition include poor feeding, vomiting, dehydration, lethargy, hypotonia, seizures, hypoglycaemia, ketoacidosis, opisthotonus, pancreatitis, coma and neurological decline.

138. D) The virus entering through whatever routes acts primarily on the following cells.

I. Lymphoreticular system
   a) CD4 + T helper cells
   b) Macrophages
   c) Monocytes
   d) B-lymphocytes

II. Certain endothelial cells

III. CNS
   b) Microglia of nervous system
   c) Astrocytes
   d) Oligodendrocytes
   e) Neurons: Indirectly by the action of cytokines and gp-120

139. D) Major hisocompatibility complex, **also known as the human leukocyte** antigen (HLA), has role in the immune responses and disease. The genes that code for the HLA antigens are found on the short arm of sixth pair of chromosome (one paternal and one maternal). The cluster of genes constitutes the human major histocompatibility (MCH) and is also known as the HLA complex. The MCH genes are contained within four HLA loci known as A, B, C, and D. There are three classes of genes in these HLA loci.

MCH class 1 molecules: In humans the genes encoding the major transplantation antigens are HLA-A, HLA-B and HLA-C loci. The products of these loci are known as class I antigen. Class one antigens are membrane bound glycoprotein in nature. They are composed of two polypeptide chains. The smaller one is known as B_2-microglobulin. The larger polypeptide chain of class I antigen is encoded by a gene present on HLA-A, HLA-B and HLA-C regions. It is known as Alpha chain and has a molecular weight of 44,ooo daltons. The globular protein formed by these two peptides is present on the surface of virtually all nucleated cells and platelets.

MCH class II molecules: Class II antigens are coaded by the HLA-DP, HLA-DQ, and HLA-DR loci. They are glycoproteins consisting of two polypeptide chains (A and B) held together by non-covalent interactions. In man they are normally found on immunologically reactive cells (monocytes, macrophages, and dendritic cells) B and T lymphocytes.

MCH class III molecules: These proteins are components of complement system (C2, C4, and properdin factor B). Cytokines TNF-a and b are also encoded within the MHC. This class of antigen does not act as histocompitability antigen.

140. D) Cells secreting leukotrienes are monocytes, basophils, neutrophils, eosinophils, mast cells, and epithelial cells.

Platelets produce thromboxane (TxA2, TxB2), Lipoxin (LxB4, LxA4).

141. D) Two types of delayed hypersensitivity reactions are recognized:

1. Tuberculin type
2. Contact dermatitis type

Immediate hypersensitivity reaction occurs in:

1. Atopy
2. Anaphylaxis

3. ABO blood transfusion reactions
4. Rh incompatibility reaction
5. Autoimmune diseases
6. Reactions against tissue antigen: Goodpasture's syndrome, Pemphigus
7. Arthus reaction
8. Serum sickness

142. A) Gaucher's disease is a heredofamilial disease due to deficiency of glucocerebrosidase. As a result, glucocerebroside accumulation principally in the reticuloendothelial cells.

Tay-Sach's disease is characterized by the increased accumulation of gangliosidosis (Gm_2) in brain and spleen.

Niemann-Pick disease is a systemic lipoidosis is characterized by the accumulation of sphingomyelin predominantly and gangliosides in small amounts in reticuloendothelial cells in visceral organs.

von-Gierke's disease type I glycogenosis resulting from the lack of glucose 6 phosphatase, is the most common example of the hepato-renal form of glycogenesis. Liver cells, kidney, cardiac muscle fibres, skeletal muscles, smooth muscles of elementary tract urinary bladder, blood vessels and b...chial cartilage cells show intracytoplasmic deposition of glycogen.

143. D) Russell bodies are eosinophilic large homogenous immunoglobulin –containing inclusions usually in plasma cells undergoing excessive synthesis of immunoglobulin; the Russell body is characteristic of the distended endoplasmic reticulum. Russell bodies are round to ovoid formations, measuring from 20 to 40 μm in diameter. They have homogenous, bright red high refractile cytoplasm with no nucleus.

Russell bodies are seen in:

1. Rhinoscleroma
2. Multiple myeloma
3. Plasmacytotma

144. B) Rhinoscleroma

The cellular infiltrate is very rich in plasma cells and lymphocytes. The characteristic cells are known as **Mikulicz cells** called after a German surgeon. Mikulicz cell is a large histiocyte measuring up to 100 um in diameter. They are filled by pale gelatinous material, giving the cytoplasm a foamy appearance and eccentric nucleus. One finds within the cytoplasm of Mikulicz cells many bacilli called Klebsiella Rhinoscleromatis offrisch bacilli. They can be visualized with Giemsa"s stain or a silver stain.

145. B) Interalveolar capillaries are distended and tortuous. The alveolar walls are thickened. More severe injury to blood vessels causes small haemorrhages, especially in the lung with escape of few R B Cs into the alveoli. Haemoglobin of disintegrated RBCs is converted into hemosiderin, when they are taken up by macrophages, which accumulate in alveoli, known as **heart failure cells**. These are septal histiocytes derived from the alveolar septa may be found in the septum. The macrophages accumulate in the alveoli around respiratory bronchioles and may appear in radiographs as a "**snow stom**" effect.

146. C) The colour of the mixture serves as a guide to the amount of sugar in the urine.

Blue colour – Sugar is absent
Green PPT – 0.5% sugar
Yellow – 1% sugar
Orange – 1.5% sugar
Brick red – 2% or more sugar

Benedict's reagent is used as a test for the presence of all monosaccharides and generally also reducing tests.

147. A) **Jaundice**: Orange colour of urine is due to dehydration, jaundice, ingestion of blackberries, beet, rhubarb and seen herb.

Pale urine in diabetes insipidus.

Reddish brown in increased haemoglobin in urine

148. A) Sarcoidosis : On X-ray – A description for the enlarged nodular hilar and mediastinal lymph nodes typical of sarcoidosis.

149. C) Xanthomatosis is a systemic lipidosis characterized by the accumulation of cholesterol in reticuloendothelial system and hyperlipidaemia. The local lesions occur in cases of hyperlipidaemias and have been given different names.

Yellowish small or fleshy nodules in subcutaneous tissue, occurring around joints has been termed xanthoma tuberosum. Similar nodules may occur in the extensor tendons of the fingers, tendons below the knee joints and in tendons in the tendo Achilles: these are tendon xanthomas and quite similar to the so-called giant cell tumour of tendon sheath.

150. A) Commonest worldwide cause of primary immunodeficiency is isolated IgA deficiency.

Patients with isolated deficiency of IgA usually present with recurrent respiratory infections. IgA deficiency frequently occurs in autoimmune disorders (systemic lupus erythematosus, rheumatoid arthritis, and coeliac disease). IgA deficient patients may form anti IgA antibodies in high titre; when such patients receive blood transfusion containing IgA, anaphylactic reaction can occur.

151. C) X-LINKED INFANTILE HYPOGAMMAGLOBULINAEMIA also referred to as Bruton's hypoglobinaemia or agammaglobulinaemia. This is the first immunodeficiency disease to have been recognized. Bruton described it in 1952. Symptoms usually arise in the first or second year of life, protection before that being provided by maternal antibodies of IgG class transmitted to the fetus. It is characterized by recurrent infection by pyogenic bacteria such as pneumococci, streptococci, and haemophilus. The most common type of infections includes sinusitis, pneumonia, otitis, furunculosis, meningitis and septicemia. Patients are also at increased risk for development of pneumocystitis carinii pneumonia. Persistent generalized infections with Giardia lamblia may give rise to malabsorption. The haemopoietic marrow contains normal numbers of pre-B cells but the lymph nodes and tonsils are small, but biopsy reveals an absence of germinal centers and plasma cells. The rectal biopsy reveals absence of plasma cells. **The patients have failure of B cell maturation associated with a defective B cell tyrosine kinase also called as Bruton tyrosine kinase (btk gene).** Because BTK maps to the X chromosome, the disorder is seen primarily in males. There is severe hypogammaglobulinaemia but serum contains some γ-globulin. **Status of cell-mediated immunity is normal but lymphoid tissue lacks B cells.**

152. C) DIGEORGE SYNDROME (Thymic hypoplasia): This is most clearly defined T cell immunodeficiency and is also known as congenital thymic aplasia/hypoplasia, or immunodeficiency with hypoparathyroidism. Thymic hypoplasia results from a congenital malformation affecting the third and fourth pharyngeal pouches. These structures give rise to the thymus, parathyroid glands, and portions of lips, ears, and aortic arch. Though del 22q11 is common, no single genetic abnormality is constant and not all babies have thymic aplasia. In those infants who survive the neonatal period, immunoglobulin production appears normal, although antibody responses are impaired, because of lack of helper T cells. **Infants with these defects are extremely vulnerable to vi-**

ral, fungal and protozoal infections and suffer from tetany. The immunodeficiency primarily involves cell-mediated immunity. The thymus dependent areas of lymph nodes and spleen are depleted of lymphocytes. **Circulating T cells are reduced in numbers.** Thymic transplantation (immunocompetent tissue) brings success in the treatment.

153. A) NK cells are somewhat larger than small lymphocytes It comprises 10% to 15% of peripheral blood lymphocytes. NK cells are large and possess azurophilic granules and are therefore called large granular lymphocytes.

Precise origin of NK cells is unknown. These so-called 3rd population lymphocytes do not express T or B cells specific surface antigen receptors or immunoglobulins.

NK cells are capable of lysing certain tumour sensitization. They are all cytotoxic for virus infected cells and to target coated with IgG antibodies.

154. D) Common causes of hypoglycaemia

- Small dates and preterm babies
- Infants of diabetic mothers
- Polycythaemia
- Hypothermia
- Sepsis
- Asphyxia
- Respiratory distress
- Deficiency of hormones—Glucagons, hGh, ACTH, epinephrine, adrenal.
- Metabolic disease—Glycogen storage disease, Maple syrup urine disease and fructose intolerance.

155. B) Antigen presenting cells are B-cells, dendritic cells, Langerhan's cells, monocytes, macrophages and in CNS microglia.

156. B) Klinefelter's syndrome is due to sex chromosomal abnormality XXY.

Dysgenesis is defined as defective or abnormal development of an organ, especially of the gonads.

X0 abnormality of chromosome is seen in Turner's syndrome. This syndrome is found in human females.

157. D) Hurler's disease is a severe form of mucopolysacchridosis (MPS). The MPS constitute a group of hereditary disorders, having in common lysosomal accumulation of upgraded glucosaminoglycan (GAG) secondary to deficiencies of specific enzymes. All but one of the MPS is marked by urinary excretion of GAG products chondroitin sulphate, keratan sulphate, dermatan sulphate, and heparan sulphate.

158. C) Haemosiderin accumulates in the cells of islands of Langerhans, to a lesser extent in the exocrine and ductular epithelium and in macrophages. There is fibrosis, which may destroy islet tissue causes diabetes mellitus. The skin developed a bronzed appearance hence the name is bronzed diabetes.

159. B) Corticosteroids suppress inflammation at all levels there by blunting this phase of healing. These agents also inhibit collagen synthesis.

160. C) Programme cell death is known as apoptosis.

Cell death is characterized by:

1. Cell shrinkage:
2. Chromatin condensation:
3. Formation of cytoplasmic blebs (buds) and apoptotic bodies (vesicles)
4. Phagocytosis of apoptotic cells

161. A) The first effect of hypoxia is on the cell's aerobic respiration, that is, oxidative phosphorylation by mitochondria; as a consequence of reduced oxygen tension, the intracellular generation of ATP is markedly reduced. The resulting depletion of ATP has widespread effects on many systems of cell.

162. B) Extensive cellulitis is known as phlegmona diffusa. Phlegmona diffusa is a somewhat rare, or less extensive inflammation of the cutaneous and subcutaneous tissue, which is closely allied to cellulitis and erysipelas.

163. D) Metastatic calcification: Metastatic calcification is a result of an increase in the level of ionic calcium in the plasma and occurs in normal soft tissues.

The level of plasma calcium is normal and deposition is due to local changes in affected tissue. This is termed dystrophic calcification.

164. D) After activation, macrophages secrete a wide variety of biological products, that if unchecked can result in the tissue injury and fibrosis characteristic of chronic inflammation. These products include:

1. Acid and neutral proteases
2. Coagulation factors and complement
3. Reactive oxygen species and NO
4. Cytokines IL-1 And TNF
5. Growth factors

165. D) Examples of granulomatous inflammation are sarcoidosis, tuberculosis, and cat-scratch disease

166. A) Use of Southern blot hybridization technique to diagnose B-cell lymphoma by detecting clonal immunoglobulin gene rearrangements in lymph node and other biopsy tissue.

There are many uses of the Southern blot. Some of these uses are listed below:

- To identify a single gene among thousands of fragments of DNA and to detect sequences of DNA in an organism's genome.
- Used in gene therapy and gene mapping.
- To analyze the genetic pattern in an organism's DNA.
- To identify gene mutations, deletions, duplications and gene rearrangements involved in diseases.
- To determine the number of copies of a particular DNA sequence presented in the genome of an organism.
- To identify related DNA sequences in the genome and to determine if there is a gene family (a group of similar genes)
- To detect certain cancers and genetic diseases such as:
  1. Monoclonal leukaemia populations
  2. Sickle cell mutations

167. D) Hypercoagulability occurs in women taking oral contraceptives.

It occurs in cases of trauma due to damage to the vascular endothelium. Damage to the intima resulting in thrombosis.

In cases of burn there is haemoconcentration, which play a part in the process of thrombosis.

Thrombosis is a common condition in heart failure, where blood flow slows down due to stagnation of veins.

168. D) Characteristic features of hypoxic irreversible injury are:

1. Irreversible injury is marked by severe mitochondrial vacuolization.
2. Alteration of lysosomes in cell injury generally appears later. Lysosomes become swollen, and after the onset of lethal injury lysosomes rupture and this event causes leakage of lysosomal enzymes at this stage
3. Intact cell membranes are essential to the maintenance of normal cell permeability and volume loss of membrane integrity causes defects in plasma membrane permeability.

169. C) Necrosis. A glassy homogenous, increased eosinophilia with moth eaten appearances in a cell which is coupled with nuclear changes pyknosis, karyolysis, and karyohexis.

170. D) Primary influences predisposes to thrombogenesis are:

1. Endothelial injury
2. Stasis of blood
3. Turbulence of blood
4. Hypercoagulability of blood

171. A) Milroy's disease is a familial disease characterized by lymphedema, commonly in legs, caused by congenital abnormalities in the lymphatic system. Disruption of the normal drainage of lymph leads to fluid accumulation and hypertrophy of soft tissues.

It is also known as Milroy's disease, Nonne-Milroy-Meige syndrome and hereditary lymphedema.

This disease is more common in women and an association with the gene FLT4 has been described.

chapter 2

Neoplasia and Cytology

1. All are the examples of tumour markers, except:
   A) Alpha fetoprotein
   B) Thyroglobulin
   C) Alpha-HCG
   D) B2-macroglobulin
2. Best screening test for carcinoma cervix in public is:
   A) Transvaginal USG
   B) Cervical cytology
   C) Colposcopy assisted biopsy
   D) Abdominal scan
3. A marker for the diagnosis of pancreatic cancer is:
   A) CA 15-3
   B) CA 19-9
   C) Alpha fetoprotein
   D) CYFRA 21-1
4. Which of the following tumours may cause elevated CEA level:
   A) Breast cancer
   B) Colorectal cancer
   C) Gastric ulcer
   D) All of the above
5. Most common occupational cancer in India is:
   A) Skin cancer
   B) Lung cancer
   C) Bladder cancer
   D) Brain cancer
6. Marker for ovarian tumour of epithelial origin is:
   A) Fibronectin
   B) Acid phosphatase
   C) CA-125
   D) LDH
7. Kaposi's sarcoma occurs with infection due to:
   A) HHV 1
   B) HHV 2
   C) HHV4
   D) HHV 8
8. Malignant tumour which never metastasize include?
   A) Basal cell carcinoma
   B) Osteoclastoma
   C) Fibrosarcoma
   D) Rhabdomyosarcoma
9. Cytogenetic translocation abnormality (Q24 Q12) is seen in:
   A) Wilm's tumour
   B) Osteogenic sarcoma
   C) Ewing's tumour
   D) Synovial sarcoma
10. Cardiac tumours in adults is:
    A) Myxoma
    B) Rhabdomyoma
    C) Leiomyoma
    D) Fibroma

11. Intracytoplasmic glycogen is seen in:
   A) Osteogenic sarcoma
   B) Wilm's tumour
   C) Ewing's tumour
   D) Basal cell carcinoma
12. All of them are benign tumours except:
   A) Myxoma
   B) Osteoblastoma
   C) Haemangioma
   D) Hepatoma
13. Asbestos does not cause?
   A) Carcinoma larynx
   B) Mesothelioma
   C) Ca salivary gland
   D) Carcinoma stomach
14. Nickel exposure is associated with which cancer
   A) Larynx
   B) Kidney
   C) Lung
   D) Nasopharynx
15. Basal cell carcinoma is prevalent in:
   A) America
   B) Japan
   C) Australia
   D) Sweden
16. Hutchinson's freckle is also known as:
   A) Basal cell carcinoma
   B) Lentigo maligna melanoma
   C) Junctional nevus
   D) Syphilitic ulcer
17. Which of the following is not a benign tumour?
   A) Fibroadenoma
   B) Leiomyoma
   C) Chorioadenoma destruens
   D) Rhabdomyoma
18. Malignant tumour arises from testis is:
   A) Wilm's tumour
   B) Ewing's tumour
   C) Retinoblastoma
   D) Seminoma
19. Malignant childhood tumour is:
   A) Multiple myeloma
   B) Embryonal Rhabdomyosarcoma
   C) Seminoma
   D) Renal cell carcinoma
20. Kangri cancer is common on
   A) Thigh
   B) Face
   C) Thorax
   D) Abdominal wall
21. Inherited cancer syndrome include all except:
   A) Retinoblastoma
   B) Neuroblastoma
   C) Xeroderma pigmentosa
   D) Familial polyposis coli
22. Rodent ulcer is:
   A) Squamous cell carcinoma
   B) Basal cell carcinoma
   C) Sebaceous carcinoma
   D) Malignant melanoma
23. Parasite causes carcinoma urinary bladder is
   A) Entaomeba histolytica
   B) Schistosoma haematobium
   C) Trichinella spiralum
   D) Trichomonas
24. In mycosis fungoides, which of the following are affected?
   A) T4 cells
   B) T8 cells
   C) Killer cells
   D) B cells
25. Burkitt's lymphoma is caused by
   A) HPV
   B) Epstein-Barr virus
   C) HHV-8 virus
   D) HSV
26. Rosettes are seen in:
   A) Wilm's tumour
   B) Ewing's tumour
   C) Seminoma
   D) Lymphoma

27. Choriostoma is:
A) Normal tissue at abnormal sites
B) Normal tissue at normal sites
C) Abnormal tissue at any sites
D) None

28. Compared with benign tumours neoplastic tumours show except:
A) Uniform hyperchromatism
B) Uniform cell mass
C) Variable shape size
D) High mitotic figure

29. Mutation in $CDKN_2A$ and CDK_4 gene occurs in:
A) Hereditary polyposis coli
B) Malignant melanoma
C) Basal cell carcinoma
D) Rhabdomyosarcoma

30. Malignant tumour shows presence of glycogen in cytoplasm are except:
A) Renal cell carcinoma
B) Ewing's tumour
C) Acinic cell tumour of salivary gland
D) Osteogenic sarcoma

31. Cancer suppressor gene is important in which malignancy?
A) Retinoblastoma
B) Malignant melanoma
C) Liver carcinoma
D) Lung cancer

32. Increased erythropoietin is produced by:
A) Multiple myeloma
B) Renal cell carcinoma
C) Meningioma
D) Small cell carcinoma lung

33. Rosettes are not seen in:
A) Ewing's tumour
B) Neuroblastoma
C) Retinoblastoma
D) Hypernephroma

34. Viruses associated with human cancer except:
A) Epstein-Barr virus
B) Human papilloma virus
C) Hepatitis A virus
D) HSV

35. Testicular tumour most sensitive to radiation?
A) Seminoma
B) Teratoma
C) Lymphoma
D) Mixed germ cell tumour

36. Person working in vinyl chloride industries are more prone to:
A) Squamous cell carcinoma
B) Melanoma
C) Angiosarcoma
D) Transitional cell carcinoma

37. In Burkitt's lymphoma trans location is seen in chromosome:
A) 8-14
B) 15-17
C) 4-11
D) 11-14

38. Which malignancy is more common in Down's syndrome:
A) Retinoblastoma
B) Neuroblastoma
C) Non-Hodgkin's lymphoma
D) Leukaemia

39. With regard to TP53 tumour suppressor gene. Choose correct answer:
A) It is located on chromosome 17
B) It encodes 53Kda protein
C) It is stimulated by ionizing radiation
D) All of the above

40. Gene which prevents neoplasia is
A) TP 53
B) BCL2
C) NF-1 gene
D) Rb gene

41. Malignant tumours showing chromosomal abnormalities are except:
A) Burkitt's lymphoma
B) Retinoblastoma
C) Renal cell carcinoma
D) Oat cell carcinoma lung

42. Most common sarcoma in children is:
A) Fibrosarcoma
B) Embryonal rhabdomyosarcoma
C) Liposarcoma
D) Leiomyosarcoma

43. Which does not predispose to malignancy:
A) Turner's syndrome
B) Cri-du-chat syndrome
C) Down's syndrome
D) Klinefelter syndrome

44. All are increased incidence of malignancy except:
A) Down's syndrome
B) Fragile X-syndrome
C) Bloom's syndrome
D) Fanconi's anaemia

45. Viruses associated with human cancer except:
A) Herpes zoster
B) Hepatitis B virus
C) Human papilloma virus
D) Epstein-Barr virus

46. Koilocytes are seen in smear:
A) Human papilloma virus
B) Herpes virus infection
C) Gardnerella vaginalis
D) Tuberculosis

47. Cervicovaginal smears can diagnose:
A) Condyloma of the cervix
B) Fungal infection
C) Squamous cell carcinoma
D) All of the above

48. Which of the following malignant tumour is radioresistant:
A) Ewing's sarcoma
B) Retinoblastoma
C) Osteosarcoma
D) Neuroblastoma

49. Alveolar soft part sarcoma frequently originates in:
A) Chest wall
B) Head and neck
C) Retroperitoneum
D) Lower extremities

50. Most common malignant tumour in adults is:
A) Fibrosarcoma
B) Liposarcoma
C) Leiomyosarcoma
D) Rhabdomyosarcoma

51. Oral cytological smears are of no value in the diagnosis of:
A) Oral cancer
B) Primary intraoral herpes simplex
C) Herpes zoster
D) Lipoma

52. Starry sky appearance is found in:
A) Burkitt's lymphoma
B) Mycosis fungoides
C) AML
D) Sarcoidosis

53. Which of the following types of cancers are most common in organ transplantation:
A) Breast cancer
B) Lung cancer
C) Skin cancer
D) Prostate cancer

54. Which statement is not true for exfoliative cytology:
A) Extensively used mass screening of carcinoma
B) Slow but accurate procedure
C) It is not substitute but an adjunct to biopsy
D) Painless, bloodless procedure

55. Commonest site of extra-medullary plasmacytoma
A) Gums
B) Nasal cavity
C) Kidney
D) Soft tissues

56. Mantle cell lymphomas are positive for all the following except:
A) CD 23
B) CD 20
C) CD 5
D) CD 43

57. In which variant of Hodgkin's disease lacunar cell is present:
A) Nodular sclerosis
B) Lymphocytic predominance
C) Mixed cellularity
D) Lymphocytic depletion

58. In oncocytoma, the eosinophilic appearance of cell is due to presence of
A) Lysosomes
B) Enlarged mitochondria
C) Smooth endoplasmic reticulum
D) Fat

59. B-cell lymphomas do not include.
A) Small cell lymphoma
B) Follicular lymphoma
C) Cutaneous lymphoma
D) Plasmacytoid lymphoma

60. The type of lymphoma more common in females is:
A) Lymphocytic predominance
B) Lymphocytic depletion
C) Nodular sclerosing
D) Mantle cell lymphoma

61. Most commonly affected organ in MALT lymphoma is:
A) Stomach
B) Thyroid
C) Salivary gland
D) Lungs

62. Which of the liver tumour occurs in infancy?
A) Fibrolamellar carcinoma
B) Hepatoblastoma
C) Epithelial haemangioendothelioma
D) All of the above

63. Which of the following is retroperitoneal tumour:
A) Melanoma
B) Lymphoma
C) Liposarcoma
D) Adenocarcinoma

64. Which of the following lung cancer is associated with worst prognosis:
A) Small cell carcinoma
B) Adenocarcinoma
C) Alveolar carcinoma
D) Squamous cell carcinoma

65. Which of the following is the most common predisposing factor for adenocarcinoma of the oesophagus?
A) Exposure to nitrosamine
B) Gastro-oesophageal reflux disease
C) Human papilloma virus infection
D) Smoking and Tyrosis palmaris

66. The most common lung cancer seen in non-smokers
A) Small cell carcinoma
B) Large cell carcinoma
C) Adenocarcinoma
D) Squamous cell carcinoma

67. Which of the following microscopic findings, which is most likely to indicate that tumour is malignant:
A) Pleomorphism
B) Invasion
C) Atypia
D) Increased nuclear/cytoplasmic ratio

68. Deletion of Rb gene occurs in:
A) ID carcinoma
B) Cerebral astrocytoma
C) Chronic myeloid leukaemia
D) Retinoblastoma

69. Helicobactor pylori causes following lesions except:
A) Chronic gastritis
B) Carcinoma stomach
C) MALTOMA
D) Leiomyosarcoma

70. AGNOR count suggest possibility of:
A) Inflammation
B) Malignancy
C) Necrosis
D) Apoptosis

71. Which type of sarcoma has worst prognosis?
A) Liposarcoma
B) Rhabdomyosarcoma
C) Kaposi's sarcoma
D) Fibrosarcoma

72. Best prognosis in Hodgkin's disease is in:
A) Nodular sclerosis
B) Mixed cellularity
C) Lymphocytic predominance
D) Lymphocytic depletion

73. Tumours of endothelial origin includes all except:
A) Haemangioma
B) Chordoma
C) Kaposi's sarcoma
D) Haemangioendothelioma

74. Common anterior mediastinal tumour are all/ except
A) Thymoma
B) Teratoma
C) Neurogenic tumour
D) Lymphoma

75. Squamous metaplasia occurs in:
A) Colon
B) Renal pelvis
C) Prostate
D) Pulmonary alveoli

76. Which of the following forms of molecular analysis is most useful to identify in carcinogenesis?
A) FISH
B) Flow cytometry
C) Single nucleotide polymorphism
D) Tumour marker expression

77. Multiple basal cell carcinoma is a feature of :
A) Gardner's syndrome
B) Gorlin's syndrome
C) Cowden's syndrome
D) Muir-Torre syndrome

78. Familial colorectal polyposis is seen in:
A) Gorlin's syndrome
B) Cowden's syndrome
C) Gardner's syndrome
D) Xeroderma pigmentosa

79. Mutation of which gene occurs in Gardner's syndrome?
A) PTEN gene
B) APC gene
C) PTCH gene
D) MSH2

80. Multiple hamartomas are seen in:
A) Gorlin syndrome
B) Cowden's syndrome
C) Gardner's syndrome
D) Muir-Torre syndrome

81. S-100 protein antigen is associated with:
A) Melanoma
B) Squamous cell carcinoma
C) Sarcoma
D) Lymphoma

82. Benign tumour recurs after excision is:
A) Fibroma
B) Pleomorphic adenoma of salivary gland
C) Fibroadenoma breast
D) Neurofibroma

83. Lamber-Eaton myasthenia syndrome is associated with:
A) Seminoma
B) Hepatocellular carcinoma
C) Carcinoma lung
D) Gliomas

84. Occult metastases is seen in bone except:
A) Melanoma
B) Carcinoma thyroid
C) Carcinoma kidney
D) Carcinoma breast

85. Sturge-Weber syndrome is associated with:
A) Neovascular haemangioma
B) Meningeal haemangioma
C) Optic glioma
D) Cavernous haemangioma

86. HPV altered epithelial cells, perinuclear spaces and nuclear pyknosis is called as:
A) Koilocytes
B) Molluscum bodies
C) Inclusion bodies
D) Antoni A bodies

87. A developmental cyst of orofacial region occurring in neck is:
A) Thyroglossal duct cyst
B) Nasopalatine duct cyst

C) Epidermoid cyst
D) Dermoid cyst

88. A rare disorder that is characterized by non-cancerous benign growth in lymph node tissue is:
A) Reactive lymphoid aggregate
B) Castleman tumour
C) Angiolymphoid hyperplasia with eosinophils
D) Kimura's disease

89. Excessive formation of scar tissue is called:
A) Fibroma
B) Myxoma
C) Keloid
D) Myoma

90. Which stain is used to differentiate leiomyoma from fibroma?
A) PTAH stain
B) Masson's trichrome
C) Reticulin
D) Methyl green pyronin

91. The most common histological variant of liposarcoma is:
A) Round cell type
B) Pleomorphic type
C) Myxoid type
D) Sclerosing type

92. The granules seen in the granular cell myoblastoma is most likely to be:
A) Mitochondria
B) Lysosomal aggregates
C) Inclusion bodies
D) Enamel proteins

93. Chemical carcinogen, aflatoxin B_1 derived from a fungus, which contaminates grain foods most commonly induces:
A) Adenocarcinoma
B) Squamous cell carcinoma of skin
C) Hepatocellular carcinoma
D) Renal cell carcinoma

94. Highest incidence of nasopharyngeal cancer is in:
A) Indians
B) Pakistanis
C) Americans
D) Chinese

95. Cystic hygroma is:
A) Lymphangiectasia
B) Cavernous haemangioma
C) Sebaceous cyst
D) Dermoid cyst

96. Cytokeratin 5.2 is a marker of:
A) Neurofibroma
B) Carcinoma of cervix
C) Fibroid uterus
D) Rhabdomyosarcoma

97. Workers of dye industry are prone to develop carcinoma of:
A) Liver
B) Lung
C) Urinary bladder
D) Kidney

98. Exfoliative cytology is useful for diagnosis of all/E
A) Meningioma
B) Bronchial cancer
C) Cervical cancer
D) Vesical cancer

99. Tumour, which is locally malignant is:
A) Melanoma
B) Marjolin ulcer
C) Rodent ulcer
D) Osteoclastoma

100. Following tumours are benign except:
A) Papilloma
B) Seminoma
C) Fibroma
D) Rhabdomyoma

101. All are tumour markers except:
A) PSA
B) CA-125
C) Alpha-fetoprotein
D) C reactive protein

102. Exfoliative cytology is useful for the diagnosis of all/E
   A) Ca urinary bladder
   B) Thyroid
   C) Bronchial carcinoma
   D) Cervical cancer

103. Embryonic malignant tumour of infancy include all / except
   A) Neuroblastoma
   B) Medulloblastoma
   C) Nephroblastoma
   D) Osteogenic sarcoma

104. Following tumours are malignant except:
   A) Seminoma
   B) Multiple myeloma
   C) Wilm's tumour
   D) Rhabdomyoma

105. Following are tumours of first decade of life except:
   A) Retinoblastoma
   B) Neuroblastoma
   C) Rhabdomyosarcoma
   D) Ameloblastoma

106. Following tumours may produce hormones except:
   A) Choriocarcinoma
   B) Fibroma ovary
   C) Islets cell tumours of pancreas
   D) Chromophobe adenoma

107. EB virus causes all/EXCEPT
   A) Burkitt's lymphoma
   B) Nasopharyngeal carcinoma
   C) Infectious mononucleosis
   D) Carcinoma cervix

108. Tumour marker is:
   A) CM-MB
   B) C reactive protein
   C) ALT
   D) Alpha feto protein

109. Commonest malignancy seen in AIDS patient is:
   A) B-cell lymphoma
   B) Burkitt's lymphoma
   C) Kaposi's sarcoma
   D) Leukaemia

110. Potato tumour in neck is:
   A) Rhabdomyosarcoma
   B) Haemangioendothelioma
   C) Paraganglioma
   D) Mixed salivary gland tunour

111. Which tumour is not known to regress spontaneously?
   A) Choriocarcinoma
   B) Retinoblastoma
   C) Osteogenic sarcoma
   D) Melanoma

112. Exfoliative cytological smears are fixed using:
   A) Flame or heat fixation
   B) Formalin fixation
   C) Alcohol fixation
   D) Left to dry

113. The most common areas of body susceptible to carcinomas:
   A) Head and neck
   B) Back
   C) Pelvis and urogenital
   D) Extremities

114. Examples of oncofetal antigen is/are:
   A) α-fetoprotein
   B) Carcinoembryonic antigen
   C) A&B
   D) None of the above

115. A simple bacterial test for mutagenic carcinogens is:
   A) Ames test
   B) Redon test
   C) Bacteriophage
   D) Gene splicing

116. Antitumour mechanism is mediated by:
   A) Cytotoxic T lymphocytes
   B) Natural killer cells
   C) Humoral immunity
   D) All of the above

Answers

1. C) Alpha fetoprotein, thyroglobulin, and B2 macroglobulin are tumour markers. Beta HCG is a tumour marker but not an alpha HCG.

2. B) Best screening test for carcinoma cervix in public is cytological smear examination. Pap smear screening can identify potentially precancerous changes. In developed countries the widespread use of cervical screening programs has reduced the incidence of invasive cervical cancer by 50% or more.

3. B) CA 19-9 is a marker for pancreatic cancer. CA-15-3 is a marker for breast cancer. Alpha-fetoprotein is a marker for hepatocellular carcinoma and testicular cancer. CYFRA-21-1 is a marker for non-small cell carcinoma lung.

4. D) Carcinoembryonic antigen (CEA) is a glycoprotein involved in cell adhesion. It is normally produced during fetal development, but the production of CEA stops before birth. Therefore, it is not usually present in the blood in healthy adults. It was found that serum from individuals with colorectal carcinoma, gastric carcinoma, pancreatic carcinoma, lung carcinoma, and breast carcinoma as well as individuals with medullary carcinoma, had higher levels of CEA than healthy individuals.

5. A) Occupational cancers, which is common in India is skin cancers. More than 500,000 cases are diagnosed annually in India alone. Causes include, exposure to ultraviolet ray exposure at work, hyperthermia, and X-radiation in radiographers, folks that work in chemical plants or around chemicals are much more common likely to get skin cancer. Professions where people work out side are constructors, soldiers, lifeguards, policemen, and farmers. The folks are at a much higher risk of skin cancers, along folks that handle distillation and fractionation products of coal, oil shale, and petroleum.

6. C) CA-125 is an antigen present in 80% of non-mucinous ovarian carcinomas. It is defined by monoclonal antibody generated by immunizing laboratory mice with a cell line established from human ovarian carcinoma. It circulates in serum of patients with ovarian carcinoma and was therefore investigated for possible use as marker. CA 125 is often elevated with ovarian cancer, its levels, following the patient's clinical course with surgical resection or chemotherapy; the level correlates with patient response.

7. D) Kaposi's sarcoma occurs due to infection with HHV-8 virus.

8. A) Basal cell carcinoma is the most common type of skin cancer. It rarely metastasizes or kills but still it is considered malignant because it can cause significant destruction and disfigurement by invading surrounding tissues. Osteoclastoma, fibrosarcoma and rhabdomyosarcoma metastasize by blood stream.

9. C) Ewing's sarcoma and related neuroectodermal (PNET) share a unique and specific t (11.22)(q24 q12) chromosomal translocation. In Wilm's tumour mutation of the Wilm's tumour (WT1) gene locus has been reported. Synovial sarcoma is characterized by specific chromosomal translocation t (X-18)(p11 q11). Small cell osteogenic sarcoma is characterized by chromosomal translocation t (11. 22).

10. A) Myxomas are most common cardiac tumours in adults.

11. C) The Ewing's sarcoma reveals compact sheets of small polyhedral cells with pale cytoplasm and ill-defined boundaries. The nuclei are uniform, round or oval in shape, and contain scattered areas of chromatin. There are a multitude of thin walled vascular channels among a scanty stroma. The cytoplasmic material is PAS positive (glycogen) and diastase digestible. Occasional rosette or pseudorosette formation may be present.

12. D) Myxoma, haemangioma, and osteoblastoma are benign tumours. Hepatoma (hepatocellular carcinoma) is a malignant tumour arises from hepatocytes.

13. C) Exposure to asbestos can also cause laryngeal, colon and stomach cancer. Cancer of the lung occurs seven times more frequently in asbestosis. Mesothelioma of pleura and peritoneum is associated with asbestos exposure.

14. A) Carcinoma larynx is caused by exposure to nickel.

15. C) Skin cancers are the most frequently diagnosed cancers in Australia. Of these 80% are basal cell carcinoma.

16. B) Lentigo maligna melanoma represents 5% to 10% of all cases of melanoma. It occurs on the damaged skin of face in elderly people. It arises from a brown macular lesion called lentigo maligna or Hutchinson's freckle. The lesion is brown with some variation in epidermal pigment density. It has got predilection for exposed parts. As the disease advances, invasion and metastasis are frequent.

17. C) (Chorioadenoma destruens)

If a hydatidiform mole invades the myometrium, blood vessels or extends beyond the uterus, it is called invasive mole. Invasive mole shows abnormal penetration through the muscle layers of the uterus and uterine rupture may occur. Permeation in invasive mole may be extensive and may lead to persistent hæmorrhage, but serosa is usually intact.

Metastasis is often confined to the blood vessel without invasion of the surrounding tissues. Some tumour spread to the vagina, vulva, or broad ligament. Villi may embolize to distant sites-commonly in lung.

18. D) It is the commonest of malignant tumour of the testis. Seminoma make up to 30% to 40 % of all testicular tumours. Peak incidence is between 30 and 45 years. Wilm's tumour arises from kidney. Retinoblastoma is a malignant tumour of retinal anlage and Ewing's tumour is a malignant tumour of bone.

19. B) Multiple myeloma, seminoma and renal cell carcinoma occur in old age, mostly at the age of 60 years.

Embyronal rhabdomyosarcoma arises from unsegmented and undifferentiated mesoderm and is common in the head and neck region, retroperitoneum, bile ducts and urogenital tract. It is most common type, especially in children under 1 year of age. Boys and girls are equally affected. The commonest sites are vagina, urethra, bladder, prostate, epidydimis and spermatic cord.

Clinically, the tumour presents as grape like polypoidal growths protruding out of the genital tract.

20. D) Kangri cancer develop in the region of midabdomen, which gets exposed to the severe heat being generated from Kangri, which they carry around to warm off heat. Kangri cancer is peculiar in Kashmir region as the people of all age groups are accustomed to warm their bodies by the use of Kangri Baskets. This is mostly among the "not well-to do-families" who have no other means of fighting the extreme cold during winter. The ulcers are the result of continuous contact of hot pot, made up of mud enclosed in a basket made up of willow. Squamous cell carcinoma of the skin at the site of the constant heat application exists at times without lymph nodes.

21. C) Xeroderma pigmentosum is not a hereditary cancer syndrome. It is an autosomal recessive genetic disorder of DNA repair in which the ability to repair damage caused by ultraviolet light is deficient.

Multiple basal carcinomas and other skin malignancies frequently occur at an early age in those with xeroderma. Oncogene is not related with this disease

TABLE 2.1: Showing inherited cancers and related genes

No.	Inherited cancer	Abnormal gene	Other non-inherited cancers seen with this gene
1.	Retinoblastoma	RB1	Osteosarcoma
2.	Li-Fraumeni syndrome (sarcomas, Brain tumours, Leukemia)	TP53	Cancer colon and breast
3.	Melanoma	Ink4a	
4.	Colorectal cancer due to familial polyposis	APC	Most colorectal cancers
5.	Colorectal cancer without polyposis	MLH1, MSH2 or MSH6	Colorectal gastric endometrial cancers
6.	Breast and/or ovarian	BRCA1, BRCA2	Only rare ovarian cancers
7.	Wilm's tumour	WT1	Wilm's tumour
8.	Nerve tumours Including brain	NF1, NF2	Small numbers of colon cancers,melanomas
9.	Kidney cancer	VHL	Neuroblastoma, certain types of Kidney tumours

22. B) Rodent ulcer (also known as Jacob's ulcer) is a large skin lesion of nodular basal cell carcinoma. A basal cell carcinoma usually appears as a painless nodule, which develops into an equally painless ulcer. The ulcer tends to have heaped up edges with a glistening pearly appearance and nearby there are often a prominent cluster of small blood vessels. If left untreated, basal cell carcinoma enlarges and bleeds. It spreads by eating slowly into the underlying surrounding tissues; hence the name is rodent ulcer.

23. B) Carcinoma of urinary bladder is the most common malignancy in the Middle East and parts of Africa where schistosomiasis is a widespread problem. Much evidence supports the association between schistosomiasis and bladder cancer.

24. A) Mycosis fungoides (also known as Albert-Bazin-Bazin syndrome or granuloma fungoides) is the most common form of cutaneous T cell lymphoma. The disease is an unusual expression of CD4 cells immune system. It initially affects the skin, but may progress internally overtime. The disease is typically slowly progressive and chronic. In individuals with mycosis fungoides, the skin becomes infiltrated with plaques and nodules that are composed of lymphocytes. In advanced cases, ulcerated tumours and infiltration of lymph nodes by diseased cells may occur. The disorder may spread to other parts of the body, including the gastrointestinal system, liver, spleen, or brain.

25. B) Epstein-Barr virus causes Burkitt's lymphoma.

26. B) Rosette is an ornament is usually made of material gathered or pleated so as to resemble a rose and worn badge of office as evidence of won a decoration or as trimming. Rosettes are seen in Ewing's tumour. Sheets of lobules of small round cells with a scarce cytoplasm, cells are often arranged in rosettes with a neurofibrillar center. Other tumours showing rosettes are medulloblastoma, retinoblastoma, and neuroblastoma.

27. A) Choristoma is defined as a mass of histologically normal tissue in an abnormal location.

28. B) Malignant tumours show hyperchromatosis, increase mitosis, and variable cell size. Benign tumours show uniform cell mass.

29. B) In some cases developing melanoma runs in families where a mutation in the CDN 2A gene on chromosome 9 can underlie susceptibility to melanoma. Another mutation in the same gene results in a nonfunctional inhibitor of CDK4, a cyclic dependent kinase) that promotes cell division. Mutations in APC gene cause both classic and attenuated familial adenomatous polyposis. Basal cell carcinoma (basal cell nevus syndrome) is a mutation in the PTCH 1 tumour suppressor gene at chromosome 9q22.3.

Rhabdomyomas have some type of chromosomal abnormality in the cells of the tumour, which are responsible for the tumour formation. In children with an embryonal rhabdomyosarcoma there is usually an abnormality of chromosome # 11. In alveolar rhabdomyosarcoma, a rearrangement of the chromosome material between chromosome #2 and #3 is usually present. The rearrangement changes the position and functions of genes, causing a fusion of genes referred to as a "fusion transcript". Patients have an abnormal fusion transcript involving two genes known as PAX3 and FKHR.

30. D) Renal cell carcinoma, Ewing's tumour and acinic cell tumour of salivary glands shows presence of glycogen in the cytoplasm of malignant cells. Other malignant tumours with clear cytoplasm due to presence of glycogen in cell cytoplasm are clear cell carcinoma breast, dysgerminoma ovary, yolk sac tumour and endometriod tumour.

31. A) Tumour suppressor gene, or anti-oncogene, is a gene that protects the cell from one step on the path to cancer. When this gene is mutated to cause a loss or reduction in its function, the cell can progress to cancer, usually in combination with other genetic changes. Rb tumour suppressor gene is related with retinoblastoma.

32. B) Granular cell variety of renal cell carcinoma produces erythropoietin. Due to increased level of erythropoietin there is polycythaemia. Other tumours showing increased erythropoietin include, hepatocellular carcinoma, haemangioblastoma, adrenal tumours, Wilm's tumour and leiomyoma.

33. D) Rosettes are not seen in hypernephroma.

34. C) Hepatitis B not A is associated with cancer. Oncogenic viruses include Epstein-Barr virus, human papilloma virus, Herpes virus, human T cell lymphoma virus, hepatitis B virus, and hepatitis C virus.

35. A) Radiation is a common treatment for seminomas at all stages of the disease. Seminomas are sensitive to radiation therapy. NHL lymphoma is usually treated by chemotherapy. Radiation is never used as a primary therapy for non-seminoma tumours of testis.

36. C) Vinyl chloride is a toxic chemical compound frequently used in plastic industries. A known human carcinogen, vinyl chloride can cause angiosarcoma of liver, hepatocellular carcinoma, brain cancer and carcinoma lung.

37. A) Burkitt's lymphoma is due to characteristic chromosomal translocation usually t (8:14).

38. D) Leukaemia is more common in children with Down's syndrome, being seen anywhere from 10-30 times more often than in general population of children. Excluding the risk for leukaemia, the people with Down's syndrome are known to have lower risk of cancer than the general population.

39. D) Biological properties of P53 gene.

1. P53 (also known as protein 53) is a tumour suppressor protein that is encoded by TP 53 gene.
2. P53 acts as a tumour that involved in preventing cancer.
3. TP 53 is described as "the guardian of the genome", "the guardian angel gene" and the master watchman" referring to its role in conserving stability by preventing genome mutation.

4. P53 is usually found in minute quantities inside most normal cells but ionizing radiation, ultraviolet radiation, or other DNA damaging agents through post-transcription mechanisms can induce its amounts.

5. The nuclear phosphoprotein P53 functions in cell-cycle arrest, programmed cell death (apoptosis), inhibition of tumour growth and preservation of genetic stability.

6. A mutation in P53 tumour suppressor gene is found in 50% of human tumours including 60% of lung cancers. Among the other tumours involved are breast, colon, liver, prostate, bladder and skin.

40. A) The gene which prevents neoplasia is P53 gene.

41. C) Burkitt's lymphoma is due to characteristic translocation usually t (8:14). Two mutations are required to produce retinoblastoma. These involve the Rb gene, located on chromosome 13q14. The most common molecular abnormality in small cell carcinoma lung is deletion of part of chromosome 3 (3p14).

42. B) Fibrosarcoma occurs in adults. Average age is 35-55 years. Leiomyosarcoma is a disease of middle-aged persons with average age on presentation falling between fifth and sixth decades of life. In adults liposarcoma is most common presentation. Embryonal rhabdomyosarcoma is common in children.

43. B) Cri-du-chat syndrome, also known as 5p deletion syndrome, 5p minus syndrome, or Lejeune syndrome, is a rare genetic disorder due to a missing part of chromosome 5. Lejeune first described it in 1983. Leukaemia is more common in children with Down's syndrome.

Especially in mosaic cases of Turner's syndrome that contains Y chromosome 45, XO/ 46XY. Turner's syndrome is associated with ovarian malignancy (most common gonadoblastoma), malignant lymphoma and carcinoma colon. Patients with Klinefelter's syndrome are associated with malignant lymphoma, and acute leukaemia.

44. B) Bloom syndrome also known as Bloom-Torre-Machacek syndrome is a rare autosomal recessive chromosomal disorder characterized by a high frequency of breaks and rearrangements in an affected person's chromosomes. Dermatologist Dr David Bloom in 1954 discovered the condition. The greatly elevated rate of mutation in Bloom syndrome results in a high risk of cancer in affected individuals. Patients are predisposed to leukaemias, lymphoma and Fanconi's anaemia is a genetic disease that affects children and adults from all ethnic backgrounds. Many patients eventually develop acute myelogenous leukaemia, oesophageal, gastrointestinal and vulvar carcinoma. Leukaemia is more common in children with Down's syndrome.

45. A) Hepatitis B virus is associated with hepatocellular carcinoma. Epstein-Barr virus is a human herpes virus discovered in 1964, implicated in Burkitt's lymphoma, nasopharyngeal carcinoma, Hodgkin's lymphoma, B cell lymphoma, immuno-blastic lymphoma, and primary central nervous system lymphoma.

46. A) Koilocytes are type of dysplastic squamous cells found in potentially precancerous lesions. They have characteristics:

- Nuclear enlargement (two to three times normal)
- Irregularity in nuclear contour
- Hyperchromasia
- Perinuclear clearing
- The changes occur in the presence of human papilloma virus infection.

47. D) Cervicovaginal smear can diagnose hormonal changes in endometrium, inflammation, (tubercular, trichomonas, fungal, condyloma (human papilloma virus infection), filarial, Gardnerella vaginalis, dysplasia, and malignancy.

48. C) Tumours, which are sensitive to radiation include: Ewing's tumour, retinoblastoma, and neuroblastoma.

49. D) Alveolar rhabdomyosarcoma occurs in adolescents and young adults, most often females. It is well-circumscribed and encapsulated tumour of the lower extremities often arising in the mid-thigh region.

50. B) Malignant tumour commonest in adults is liposarcoma.

51. D) In cases of lipoma of oral cavity fine needle aspiration is preferable. Oral cytological smears are useful in cases of oral cancers, primary intraoral herpes simplex and herpes zoster.

52. A) The tumour cell exhibits a diffuse, almost coherent pattern, is a little larger than small lymphocytes (10-25 μm), round, nuclei with several prominent basophilic nucleoli and has a high nuclear/ cytoplasmic ratio. Chromatin is coarse with thick nuclear membrane and numerous mitoses. In most patients, non-neoplastic macrophages with abundant, pale cytoplasm are scattered among the tumours. Cytoplasm is amphophilic and strongly pyronophilic. Often they contain phagocytosed debris of tumour cells. The pale macrophages scattered among the dark tumour cells give the lesion a *starry sky appearance*, often striking in Burkitt's lymphoma.

53. C) Organ transplant recipients are particularly more prone to skin cancers. Up to 70% of recipients will develop skin cancer within 20 years of transplant. Skin cancer development occurs as much younger age in transplant recipients, as much as 20-40 years before the general population. Squamous cell carcinoma is 65 times more likely in organ transplant recipients. Basal cell carcinoma is 10 times more likely in organ transplant recipient. Melanoma is 3 times more likely in organ transplant recipients.

54. B) It is rapid procedure but not accurate because of false negative results.

55. B) 80% of extramedullary plasmacytoma occurs in soft tissues such as paranasal sinuses and nasal cavity.

56. D) Immunophenotype profile consists of C20, and CD5, (80%) CD 23.

57. A) In some Reed-Sternberg cell variant the cytoplasm shrinks during formalin fixation and processing of tissue, leaving an empty space around the nucleus. Such Reed-Sternberg variants are known as lacunar cells. Lacunar cell primarily associated with nodular sclerosis type of Hodgkin's disease.

58. B) The oncocytoma is an epithelial tumour composed of oncocytes, large eosinophilic cells having small, round, benign appearing nuclei with large nucleoli. Sheets of large swollen polyhedral oncocytes, which are granular acidophilic cells with centrally located nuclei, mark the histology. The granules are created by mitochondria.

59. C) Cutaneous lymphoma is T-cell lymphoma. Precursor B cell neoplasm

- Precursor B –lymphoblastic lymphoma-leukemia

Mature (peripheral) B-cell lymphoma

1. B-cell small lymphocytic lymphoma
2. Lymphoplasmacytic lymphoma

- Splenic marginal zone lymphoma

1. Plasma cell myeloma/ plasmacytoma
2. Extranodal marginal zone B-cell lymphoma of MALT type
3. Nodal marginal zone B-cell lymphoma (with or without monocytoid B cell)
4. Follicular lymphoma
5. Mantle cell lymphoma
6. Diffuse large B- cell lymphoma
7. Burkitt's lymphoma

60. C) Lymphocytic predominance, lymphocytic depletion and mantle cell lymphoma are common in males. Nodular sclerosing Hodgkin's lymphoma is slightly more common in females.

61. A) MALT lymphoma is a relatively rare form of non-Hodgkin's lymphoma. MALT lymphoma starts in mucosa associated lymphoid tissue that is found in other parts of body such as stomach, thyroid gland, salivary glands, and eyes, therefore known as extranodal lymphoma. The mostly affected organ is stomach.

62. B) The liver tumour occurs in infancy is hepatoblastoma. Fibrolamellar carcinoma is a tumour in adults. Epitheloid haemangioendothelioma is common in the age group 12 to 16. Other malignant tumour in infancy is hepatocellular carcinoma.

63. C) Malignant retroperitoneal tumour is liposarcoma.

64. A) Prognostic factors in non-small cell carcinoma of lung cancer include presence or absence of pulmonary symptoms, tumour size, cell type, degree of spread, and metastases to multiple lymph nodes and vascular invasion. For all small cells lung carcinoma prognosis is also generally poor. The overall five years survival for patients with SCLC is about 5%. Patients with extensive stage SCLC have an average five-year survival rate of less than 1%. The median survival time for limited stage disease is 20 months, with a five years survival rate of 20%.

65. B) Gastrointestinal reflux disease (GERD) and its resultant Barrett's oesophagus increase oesophageal cancer risk due to the chronic irritation of the mucosal lining. Adenocarcinoma is more common in this condition, while other risk factors predispose more for squamous cell carcinoma. Predisposing factors for squamous cell oesophageal carcinoma are human papilloma virus, nitrosamine, tobacco, smoking, Plummer-Vinson's syndrome, Tylosis and Howel-Evan's syndrome, Coeliac disease, alcohol consumption and achalasia.

66. A) Occurrence of lung cancer in non-smokers, who account for 15% of cases, is often attributed to a combination of genetic factors, radon gas, asbestos, viral infection and air pollution including second-hand smokers. Most common lung cancer seen in non-smokers is small cell carcinoma.

67. B) Pleomorphism, atypia and increased nuclear/cytoplasmic ratio are features of dysplasia. Invasion of surrounding tissues, nerves and blood vessels are features of malignancy.

68. D) **Rb gene**: The Rb gene is a well-known tumour suppressor gene located at 13 q14.11, and is deleted in the germ-line in one half of chromosome the child inherits in familial retinoblastoma. Afterwards it was found that apart from retinoblastoma homozygous loss of this gene was fairly common in osteosarcoma, pineal/supraseller/paraseller intracranial retinoblastoma.

69. D) Helicobacter pylori is now suspected of causing stomach cancer. It causes chronic antral gastritis which when becomes atrophic, followed by intestinal metaplasia of lining cells, dysplasia, predisposes to cancer. Helicobacter pylori is able to reduce preservative nitrates to carcinogenic nitrites. B cell lymphomas of the mucosa associated lymphoid tissue arise in the gastrointestinal epithelium as a result of T cell stimulation. The T cells are set off by Helicobacter pylori infection. The gastric lymphomas are of B cell origin, and because the transformed B cells normally reside in the marginal zones of lymphoid follicles; these tumors are also called MALTomas (marginal zone- associated lymphomas).

70. B) AgNOR counts: This is a recent technique for indirect evidence of malignancy. In every nucleus, near the nucleolus are located minute strands of generic ribosome proteins. This structure is known as "Nucleolar Organiser Region" or NOR. This structure can be specifically stained as one or more black dots by silver stains (silver = Ag), hence complex is called AgNOR. The number of AgNOR dots increases as the cells multiply and the number is an indication of proliferation of cells. Counting the AgNOR in section or smears is therefore an indication of possible neoplasia.

71. B) Rhabdomyosarcoma have very poor prognosis.

Leiomyosarcoma has a good prognosis unless it is in the gastrointestinal tract.

Liposarcomas have good prognosis if completely removed.

Fibrosarcoma have a survival rare of 60%

72. C) The prognosis can also be correlated with the histological type. In general, the outlook is most favourable when lymphocytes are abundant and Reed-Sternberg and Hodgkin's cells sparse. Thus lymphocyte-predominant type is associated with a much longer survival than the lymphocyte-depleted type, while mixed-cellularity type has an intermediate prognosis.

73. B) Chordoma arises from notochordal remnants, and usually develops within or in close proximity to the axial skeleton. Chordomas originate from the embryonic vestiges of the notochord represented by the nucleus pulposes of the intervertebral discs.

Clinically: Chordoma usually comes to notice in adult life (fifth to seventh decade) and most commonly involves the sacrococcygeal region and sphenooccipital part of the skull base. Chordoma in the sacrum and coccyx may present as low back pain and tenderness, or with symptoms of obstruction such as constipation or painful bowel movements.

Gross: The tumour is soft, almost translucent and gelatinous.

Microscopically: The tumour forms lobulated masses with large, clear, closely packed polyhedral, physalliferous cells, and strands of fibrous tissue containing blood vessels. The cells are distended with mucous material with vacuolated cytoplasm.

They are locally invasive and carry a poor prognosis despite benign histological appearances.

Chordomas are relatively radio-resistant, requiring high doses of radiation to be controlled.

On plain X-ray chordomas appear as a solitary mid-line lesion with bony destruction. There is often an accompanying soft tissue mass.

74. C) Neurogenic tumours are present in posterior mediastinum.

Anterior mediastinal tumours include:

- Thymoma
- Thymic carcinoma
- Thymic carcinoid
- Thymolipoma
- Teratoma
- Lymphoma
- Primary germ cell tumour
- Lymphangioma
- Parathyroid adenoma
- Congenital cysts

75. B) Squamous metaplasia

1. Pseudostratified ciliated columnar epithelium of bronchus, on chronic irritation by tobacco smoke and bronchiectasis is replaced by stratified squamous epithelium. In the cervix normal columnar mucus secreting epithelium of endocervix changes to squamous epithelium in response to the acid vaginal environment in chronic inflammation in prolapse uterus.

2. Transitional epithelium of the urinary bladder and renal pelvis may under go metaplasia of squamous or mucus secreting epithelium in response to chronic irritation by bladder calculi, infection and schistosomiasis.
3. Gall bladder: Normal simple columnar epithelium is replaced by squamous epithelium in chronic cholecystitis and chronic cholelithiasis.
4. Squamous metaplasia is reasonably common in ducts of salivary glands, pancreas, in mucosa of prolapsed bowel, endometrial polyp and in chronic inflammation of prostate, epididymis and thyroid gland
5. Vitamin A deficiency causes squamous metaplasia in the nose, bronchi, urinary tract, lacrimal and salivary gland,
6. Continued irritation of serosal surface (peritoneum may also result in a change from simple squamous epithelium to cuboidal, columnar or even stratified squamous epithelium.

76. C) SNPs can be analyzed to find alterations present in cancer cells. One could analyze multiple histologically similar cancers to determine what gene(s) alteration (s) such as deletions and amplifications may underlie carcinogenesis.

Using millions of SNPs can produce virtual karyotype down to the gene level.

FISH is useful to identify abnormal expression of known genes, because a specific marker is needed.

77. B) Some or all of the following may be seen in someone with Gorlin's syndrome.

1. Multiple basal cell carcinomas of the skin.
2. Odontogenic keratocysts: Seen in 75% of patients and is the most common finding. There are multiple lesions in mandible.
3. Rib and vertebrae anomalies.
4. Intracranial calcifications.
5. Skeletal abnormalities: Bifid ribs, kyphoscoliosis, early calcification of falx cerebri.
6. Distinct facies: Frontal and temporoparietal bossing, hypertelorism and mandibular prognathism.

78. C) Gardner's syndrome, also known as familial colorectal polyposis, is an autosomal dominant form of polyposis characterized by the presence of multiple polyps in the colon together with tumours outside the colon.

Extracolonic tumours may include osteomas of the skull, thyroid cancers, epidermoid cysts, fibromas, and sebaceous cysts as well as the occurrence of desmoid tumours in approximately 15% of affected individuals.

79. B) Gardner's syndrome is now known to be caused by the mutation in the APC gene located on chromosome 5q 21 (band q 21 on chromosome 5).

Mutation in the PTEN gene cause Cowden syndrome.

80. C) Cowden's syndrome (also known as Cowden's disease) and multiple hamartoma syndrome is a rare autosomal dominant inherited disorder characterized by multiple tumour like growths called hamartomas and an increased risk of certain forms of cancer. People with Cowden's syndrome have an increased risk of developing several types of cancer including cancers of breast, thyroid, and uterus. Up to 75% have benign breast conditions such as ductal hyperplasia, intraductal papillomatosis, adenosis, lobular atrophy, fibroadenomas, and fibrocystic changes. Other malignancies associated with Cowden's syndrome include endometrial carcinoma and renal cancers.

81. A) Several membranes of S-100 protein family are useful as markers for certain tumours and epidermal differentiation.

82. B) Benign tumours, which recur after excision are:

1. Pleomorphic adenoma of salivary gland
2. Benign cystosarcoma phylloids
3. Seborrheic keratoses
4. Craniopharyngioma

83. C) Lambert-Eaton myasthenic syndrome is a rare autoimmune disorder that affects neuromuscular junction. 50% of cases have an associated small cell carcinoma lung. Lambert-Eaton myasthenia syndrome is associated with:

1. Non-small cell carcinoma lung
2. Small cell carcinoma lung
3. Carcinoma breast
4. Gastrointestinal carcinomas
5. Lymphoma
6. Ovarian cancers

84. D) Occult cancer, unknown primary: A malignancy of unknown primary site or origin that is symptomless, which manifest itself as metastasis.

Occult metastasis in bone is seen in primary carcinoma kidney, carcinoma thyroid, carcinoma lung, and carcinoma prostate.

85. B) Struge-Weber's syndrome sometimes referred to as encephalotrigeminal angiomatosis, is a rare congenital neurological and skin disorder. It is one of the phakomatoses and is often associated with portwine stains of the face, glaucoma, seizures, mental retardation and ipsilateral leptomeningeal angiomas.

86. A) Koilocytes are large cells, with clear cytoplasm and pyknotic nuclei with inconspicuous nucleoli. Koilocytosis is induced by human papilloma virus infection of the superficial epithelial cells of uterine cervix and oral mucosa.

87. A) Thyroglossal duct cysts are remnants of the embryonic thyroglossal duct that may occur anywhere from the tongue to the thyroid gland. Thyroglossal cyst is a congenital defect. Thyroglossal cyst arises out of remnants of the thyroglossal tract or duct-connecting thyroid to the tongue.

88. B) Castleman's disease is a very rare disorder characterized by non-cancerous growths (tumour that may develop in the lymph node tissue at a single site or throughout body). It is named after Benzamin Castleman.

89. C) Keloids are an over growth of scar tissue at the site of injuries. These are seen more often in Africans, Americans and Indians. Onset occurs most commonly in individuals aged 10 to-30 years. Keloid occurs from such injuries as surgical incisions, traumatic wounds, vaccination sites, burns, chickenpox, acne, or even minor scratches. Keloids often run in families. Genetic associations for the development of abnormal scar tissue have been found for HLA-B14, HLA-B21, HLABW16, HLA-B35, HLADR5, HLADQW3 and blood group A. Their excision is frequently followed by recurrences.

90. B) Masson's trichome stain differentiates leiomyoma from fibroma. Smooth muscles stains pink and fibrous tissue is green in colour.

91. C) The most common histological variant is myxoid type of liposarcoma (50%). Pleomorphic type is 25-35% and round cell variant is 10 to 20%.

92. B) The granules seen in the granular cell myoblastoma are polygonal accumulation of secondary lysosomes in the cytoplasm.

93. C) **Aflatoxin,** a product of the fungus Aspergillus flavus, which grows on improperly stored grain and nuts (including peanuts). Aflatoxin causes mutation of gene p53.

94. D) Highest incidence of nasopharyngeal carcinoma is in Chinese.

95. A) Lymphangiomas and cystic hygromas are rare benign hamartomatous lesions of lymphatic systems.

Whites appear to be affected more often than people of other races.

These are tumours consisting of well-formed lymph spaces lined by endothelium and supported by fibrous stroma.

96. B) It has been suggested that cytokeratin (CAM 5.2) is a useful marker to indicate malignant transformation and invasive potential in cervical neoplasm.

97. C) People who regularly work with certain chemicals or in certain industries have a greater risk of bladder cancer than general population. Organic chemicals called aromatic amines are particularly linked with bladder cancer. These chemicals are used in the dye industry.

98. A) Cells in cases of meningiomas do not exfoliate and cannot be demonstrated in CSF. Bronchial cancer cells exfoliate and can be demonstrated in sputum. In cases of carcinoma cervix malignant cells can be demonstrated in vaginal smear. Malignant cells in urine are present in cases of vesical malignancy

99. C) Rodent ulcer: It is also known as basal cell carcinoma. Clinically these tumours present as pearly papules, often containing prominent, dilated subepidermal blood vessels (telangiectasia). It begins as a small, pearly subcutaneous nodule, which slowly increases in size and forms an intractable ulcer with rolled out margins and mouse eaten appearance. A typical basal cell carcinoma develops as a slightly elevated or hemispherical nodule covered by a smooth or sometimes, horny epidermis. It is malignant and locally invasive and extremely destructive but never metastasizes. The tumour is likely to destroy deeper structures including cartilage and bone.

Melanoma is notorious for its unpredictable and widespread metastasis. Metastatic spread to bone, usually vertebrae, is a frequent finding in terminal disease and may be accompanied by multiple metastases to the lymph nodes, central nervous system, lungs, and liver.

Marjolin's ulcer refers to an aggressive squamous cell carcinoma presenting in an area of previously traumatized, chronically inflamed or scarred skin. They are commonly present in the context of chronic wounds including burn injuries, venous ulcers, ulcers from osteomyelitis.

Osteoclastoma: Biological behavior: Giant cell tumour is potentially malignant tumour. In 40 to 60% of them following surgical treatment there may be recurrence, infiltration into surrounding tissue and even metastasis to lung though the tumour is histologically benign. Most of osteoclastoma are cured by thorough removal; approximately 20 % recur; well under 5% are malignant or become malignant after radiotherapy and metastasize to lung.

100. B) Seminoma is a malignant tumour of testis.

Papilloma is a benign tumour arising from squamous epithelium or transitional epithelium. Fibroma is a benign tumour of fibrous tissue. Rhabdomyoma is a benign tumour arising from skeletal or cardiac muscle.

101. D) **C reactive protein (CRP)** is a protein found in the blood, the levels of which rise in response to inflammation. Recent research suggests that patients with elevated basal levels of CRP are at an increased risk of diabetes, hypertension and cardiovascular disease. It is not a tumour marker.

Alpha fetoprotein (AFP) is synthesized normally in early fetal life by yolk sac and fetal liver. Abnormal plasma elevations are encountered in adults with cancer arising principally in the liver and germ cells of the testis.

CA-125: C-A125 is not specific for epithelial ovarian cancer. Elevations have been observed in a variety of benign diseases including liver disease, endometriosis, pelvic inflammatory disease and early pregnancy. Elevated levels have been noted in other gynecological cancers e.g., Adenocarcinomas of the endometrium, endocervix, fallopian tube, non-gynaecological cancers such as pancreatic cancer, carcinoma colon, breast, and lung. One of the most important potential use for a serum tumour marker in early detection of CA125 levels.

1. **Prostate specific antigen:** PSA is found in astronomically high concentrations in the seminal plasma, where it is responsible for the semen liquefaction. Prostate specific antigen is a newly described serum marker, which may prove useful in monitoring therapy and prognosis of prostate carcinoma. The levels also may be increased in benign prostatic hyperplasia.

102. B) Fine needle aspiration cytology is done in diagnosis of carcinoma thyroid.

Bronchial cancer cells exfoliate and can be demonstrated in sputum. In cases of carcinoma cervix malignant cells can be demonstrated in vaginal smear. Malignant cells in urine are present in cases of vesical malignancy.

103. D) Osteogenic sarcoma is not a tumour of infancy nor it is an embryonic tumour.

Embryonic tumours of infancy include:

1. Neuroblastoma
2. Nephroblastoma
3. Medulloblastoma
4. Retinoblastoma
5. Hepatoblastoma
6. Orchioblastoma
7. Myoblastoma
8. Endodermal sinus tumour
9. Lipoblastoma

104. D) Rhabdomyoma is a benign tumour arises from skeletal or cardiac muscle.

Seminoma, multiple myeloma and Wilm's tumour are malignant.

105. D) Ameloblastoma is seen commonly in the fourth to the fifth decade of life. Retinoblastoma, neuroblastoma, rhabdomyosarcoma are tumours of infancy (up to the age of 1 year).

106. B) Fibroma ovary does not produce any hormone.

1. ACTH: Small cell carcinoma of lung, bronchial carcinoid, thymic carcinoid, produces ACTH like substance, which produces clinical sign and symptoms of Cushing syndrome.
2. Calcitonin: The best use of calcitonin as a tumour marker remains the monitoring of therapeutic efforts in medullary carcinoma of thyroid. The cells of diffuse endocrine or neuroendocrine system of cells for e.g., the thyroid C cells produce calcitonin.
3. Human chorionic gonadotrophin (HCG): Human chorionic gonadotrophin (HCG) is seen in patients with choriocarcinoma, hydatidiform mole, ovarian and testicular teratomas. High levels of HCG in the CSF of a patient with a known extracranial source, is indicative of a CNS metastasis.*
4. Patients with insulin producing islet cell tumours of pancreas, excessive insulin is produced in the blood that causes large decreases in blood sugar levels so that patient suffer from severe effects of blood sugar.
5. Adrenal gland tumours produce steroids, aldosterone, and catecholamines.
6. Pituitary adenoma secretes adrenocorticotrophic hormone, growth hormone, luteinising hormone and thyroid stimulating hormone.

107. D) Ebstein Barr virus: Ebstein Barr virus is a human herpes virus discovered in 1964, implicated in Burkitt's lymphoma, nasopharyngeal carcinoma, Hodgkin's disease, B cell lymphoma, immunoblastic lymphoma, natural killer cell lymphoma and primary central nervous system lymphoma in AIDS.

Carcinoma cervix is one of the important cancers is caused by HPV 16 and HPV 18.

108. D) Alpha fetoprotein (AFP) is synthesized normally in early fetal life by yolk sac and fetal liver. Abnormal plasma elevations are encountered in adults with cancer arising principally in the liver and germ cells of the testis.

Alpha-fetoprotein is a marker for hepatocellular carcinoma and testicular cancer.

109. C) HIV related malignancy: Kaposi's sarcoma is the most common malignancy associated with HIV-1 infection. Human herpes virus 8 has been proposed as a possible cause of Kaposi's sarcoma in AIDS patients.

Systemic non-Hodgkin's lymphoma and primary cerebral lymphoma usually complicates late stage of HIV.

Cervical carcinoma is also increased in patients with AIDS. This is attributable to a high prevalence of human papillomavirus infection in patients with AIDS and AIDS related immuno-compromise.

Leukaemia is also associated with AIDS.

110. C) Potato tumour is carotid body tumour or chemodectoma or paraganglioma. A paraganglioma is a rare neuroendocrinal neoplasm that may develop at various body sites (including the head, neck, thorax and abdomen).

The paraganglioma appear grossly as sharply circumscribed polypoid masses and they are highly vascular tumours and may have a deep red colour.

Chemodectoma is a rare tumour of the endocrine tissue of the carotid body. In most of the cases tumour is benign but can have a malignant behaviour.

111. C) Osteogenic sarcoma: Spontaneous regression is defined as the partial or complete disappearance of a malignant tumour in the absence of all treatment or in the presence of therapy which is considered inadequate to exert a significant influence on neoplastic disease.

Spotaneous regression occur in melanoma, neuroblastoma, retinoblastoma, lymphoma/leukaemia, Choriocarcinoma, renal cell carcinoma, infantile fibrosarcoma, clear cell carcinoma of endometrium, soft tissue sarcoma.

112. C) The smears are wet fixed in a suitable fixative for about 30 minutes. The commonly used fixatives are 90% ethyl alcohol, ether alcohol in equal proportion.

113. A) 90% of common skin tumours occur on head and neck, regions most exposed to sun whereas melanocarcinomas occur on back.

114. C) Alpha fetoprotein (AFP) is synthesized normally in early fetal life by yolk sac and fetal liver. Abnormal plasma elevations are encountered in adults with cancer arising principally in the liver and germ cells of the testis.

Alpha-fetoprotein is a marker for hepatocellular carcinoma and testicular cancer.

Carcinoembryonic antigen (CEA) is a glycoprotein involved in cell adhesion. It is normally produced during fetal development, but the production of CEA stops before birth. Therefore, it is not usually present in the blood in healthy adults. It was found that serum from individuals with colorectal carcinoma, gastric carcinoma, pancreatic carcinoma, lung carcinoma, and breast carcinoma as well as individuals with medullary carcinoma, had higher levels of CEA than healthy individuals.

115. A) A simple bacterial test for mutagenic carcinogens is Ames test.

The Ames test is a biological assay to assess the mutagenic potential of chemical compounds. A positive test indicates that the chemical is mutagenic and therefore may act as a carcinogen, since cancer is often linked to mutation.

The procedure is described by Bruce Ames in 1970. The test uses a several strains of bacterium typhimurium that carry mutations in genes involved in histidine synthesis e.g., it is an autotrophic mutant, so that they require histidine for growth.

116. D) Both cell mediated and humoral immunity plays important role in antitumour mechanism. Cytotoxic T lymphocytes-has protective role against virus associated neoplasms (Burkitt's lymphoma).

NK cells are first time of defense in all tumours. Humoral mechanisms function by inactivating the complement and induction of antigen dependent cellular activity.

chapter 3

HAEMATOLOGY

1. Heinz bodies are seen in RBCs:
   A) G6PD deficiency anaemia
   B) Pernicious anaemia
   C) Aplastic anaemia
   D) Rh incompatibility
2. Direct antiglobulin test is positive in except
   A) ABO incompatibility
   B) Autoimmune haemolytic anaemia
   C) Haemolytic uraemic syndrome
   D) Rh incompatibility in infant
3. pH of Tris EDTA boric acid buffer is
   A) 9.4
   B) 5.6
   C) 8.6
   D) 7.2
4. Characteristics of intravascular haemolysis are except:
   A) Increased haptoglobin
   B) Haemoglobinuria
   C) Haemosiderinuria
   D) Increased unconjugated bilirubin
5. Hb A_2 is increased in:
   A) α thalassaemia homozygous
   B) α thalassaemia major
   C) α thalassaemia minor
   D) Sickle cell disease
6. Bence Jones proteins are found in urine of patient with:
   A) Multiple myeloma
   B) Hodgkin's lymphoma
   C) Infectious mononucleosis
   D) Paget's disease
7. Structure of HBH is:
   A) $\alpha_2 \beta_2$
   B) $\alpha_2 \gamma_2$
   C) β_4
   D) γ_4
8. Abnormalities of blood clotting occurs in except:
   A) Patient taking brufen
   B) Christmas disease
   C) Sickle cell anaemia
   D) von-Willebrand disease
9. Howell-Jolly bodies seen in:
   A) Iron deficiency anaemia
   B) Pernicious anaemia
   C) β-Thalasaemia
   D) Aplastic anaemia
10. Hyposegmented neutrophils are seen in:
    A) CML
    B) Addison's anaemia
    C) Iron deficiency anaemia
    D) Myelodysplasias
11. Structure of HBF is:
    A) $\alpha_2 \beta_2$
    B) $\alpha_2 \gamma_2$
    C) β_4
    D) γ_4

12. Most iron is stored in combination with
A) Sulphite
B) Ferritin
C) Transferrin
D) Ascorbic acid

13. Adults with sickle cell anaemia most commonly experience neurological complications as which of the following:
A) Intracranial haemorrhage
B) Cerebral infarction
C) Seizures
D) Ataxia

14. Perinuclear halo seen in cells of multiple myeloma is due to:
A) Ribosomes number is hugely increase
B) Prominent golgi apparatus
C) Vacuolization of cells
D) Numerous mitochondria

15. Any of the following can be a cause of leukopaenia except:
A) Typhoid
B) Rhinovirus
C) Malaria
D) X-ray irradiation

16. On haemoglobin electrophoresis fastest moving abnormal haemoglobin is:
A) Haemoglobin A
B) Haemoglobin J
C) Haemoglobin H
D) Haemoglobin E

17. A 24-year-old female presents with palpable purpura and with rashes all over trunk, limbs and abdomen. The most possible diagnosis is:
A) Meningococcemia
B) Henoch-Schonlein purpura
C) Thrombocytopaenic purpura
D) Acute leukaemia

18. Haemoglobin which crosses haemoglobin A band on cellullose acetate strips are except:
A) Haemoglobin D
B) Haemoglobin J
C) Haemoglobin H
D) Haemoglobin Bart

19. Hypersegmented neutrophils are seen in:
A) Iron deficiency anaemia
B) Thalassaemia
C) Pernicious anaemia
D) Aplastic anaemia

20. Philadelphia chromosome is associated with:
A) CML
B) Adult ALL
C) All of the above
D) None of the above

21. Which of the following chronic disorder is not associated with anaemia?
A) Uremia
B) Liver disease
C) Gall bladder stone
D) Tuberculosis

22. Which of the following combination of cytogenetic abnormallity and associated leukaemia/lymphoma is incorrect?
A) t (8:14) Burkitt's lymphoma
B) t (15:17) AML-M3
C) t (9:22) CML
D) t (9:20) ALL

23. Microcytic hypochromic anaemia is not seen in:
A) Sideroblastic anaemia
B) Thalassaemia
C) Iron deficiency anaemia
D) Vitamin C deficiency anaemia

24. Microcytic hypochromic anemia is seen in:
A) Folic acid anaemia
B) Sideroblastic anaemia
C) Myelofibrosis
D) Sickle cell anaemia

25. Macrocytic hypochromic anaemia is seen in except:
A) Pernicious anaemia
B) Folic acid anaemia
C) Vitamin B_6 anaemia
D) Hypothyroidism

26. In anaemia of chronic diseases which of the following finding is incorrect:
A) Microcytic hypochromic anaemia

B) TIBC increases
C) Serum ferritin increases
D) MCHC decreases

27. MCHC is increased in:
A) Spherocytosis
B) Pernicious anaemia
C) Iron deficiency anaemia
D) Sickle cell anaemia

28. Normal M:E ratio is:
A) 9:1
B) 6:1
C) 3:1
D) 5:1

29. Blood transfusion least likely to develop:
A) AIDS
B) Syphilis
C) Hepatitis
D) Malignancy

30. What is the size of microfilter used in blood transfusion sets:
A) 50 micrometer
B) 150 micrometer
C) 170 micrometer
D) 250 micrometer

31. Which of the following is not found in cryo-precipitate:
A) Fibrinogen
B) Antithrombin
C) vWF
D) Factor VIII

32. Bone marrow iron is increased in which of the following conditions?
A) Iron deficiency anaemia
B) Thalassaemia
C) Polycythaemia
D) Leukaemia

33. ESR is increased in except:
A) Myocardial infarction
B) Tuberculosis
C) Sickle cell anaemia
D) Rheumatoid arthritis

34. Normal MCV is:
A) 110 femtoliter
B) 45 femtoliter
C) 90 femtoliter
D) 70 femtoliter

35. One unit of fresh blood rises the HB% concentration by:
A) 0.1 gram
B) 1 gram
C) 2 gram
D) 2.2 gram.

36. Blood is stored at:
A) –20ºC
B) +2ºC to +6ºC
C) –0 to 1ºC
D) –4ºC to 0ºC

37. CML is associated with all of the following except:
A) Increased platelet count
B) Anaemia
C) Increased leukocytic alkaline phosphatase
D) Increased leukocyte count

38. Poor prognostic indicator of ALL is:
A) Female sex
B) Leukocyte < 50,000
C) Age > 1 year
D) Hypodiploidy

39. Sickle cell disease is associated with all except:
A) Pripism
B) Impaired fertility in women
C) Increased incidence of stroke
D) Gall stones in majority of cases

40. Hazards of exchange transfusion are all except:
A) Oligaemic shock
B) Citrate tetany
C) Cardiac arrest
D) Hypokalemia

41. Commonest cause of aplastic anaemia is:
A) Idiopathic
B) Chloramphenicol
C) Phenylbutazone
D) Petroleum products

42. Normal Hb1C level is:
A) 11%
B) 5-6%
C) 8%
D) 9%

43. Genetic syndrome associated with childhood leukaemia except
A) Fanconi's anaemia
B) Patau's syndrome
C) Acquired immunodeficiency syndrome
D) Bloom's syndrome

44. Following condition is haemoglobinopathy
A) G6PD deficiency
B) von Willebrand disease
C) Spherocytes
D) Thalassaemia

45. Commonest cause of anaemia in childhood is:
A) Iron deficiency
B) Folic acid
C) Pyridoxine deficiency
D) Vitamin B12 deficiency

46. For acute leukaemia blast cells should be more than:
A) 10%
B) 20%
C) 30%
D) 40%

47. All of the following are true of β thalassaemia major except:
A) Microcytic hypochromic anaemia
B) Increased HBF
C) Target cells in peripheral smear
D) Increased osmotic fragility

48. 12 year old boy presented with one day history of bleeding gums, subconjunctival bleed and purpuric rash. Peripheral smear was suggestive of acute myeloid leukaemia. Which of the following is the most likely:
A) Myeloblastic leukaemia without maturation
B) Myeloblastic leukaemia with maturation
C) Promyelocytic leukaemia
D) Myelomonocytic leukaemia

49. A non-bleeding 70Kg adult is transfused with 8 units of platelets. The pre-transfusion platelet count is 70,000/mm². The expected post-transfusion platelet count should be about:
A) 80,000
B) 90,000
C) 115,000
D) 157,000

50. Hereditary spherocytosis is due to deficiency of all except:
A) Ankyrin
B) Anion exchanger transporter deficiency
C) Glycophorin 2
D) Spectrin

51. In promyelocytic leukaemia translocation is seen in chromosome:
A) T(8-14)
B) t(15-17)
C) t (12-14)
D) t(4-11)

52. Which of the following haemoglobin estimation will be diagnostically helpful in a case of beta thalassaemia trait?
A) HBF
B) Hb 1C
C) HB A_2
D) HbH

53. Autoimmune haemolytic anaemia is mostly associated with:
A) B cell lymphoma
B) T cell lymphoma
C) Histiocytosis
D) Myeloid disorders

54. In a patient with Thalassaemia peripheral blood film for cell morphology shows:
A) Macrocytosis
B) Normocytic normochromic anaemia
C) Microcytic hypochromic RBCs
D) Spherocytosis

55. Microangiopathic haemolytic anaemia occurs in:
A) DIC

B) Haemolytic uremic syndrome
C) Disseminated malignancy
D) All of the above

56. Commonest type of ALL is:
A) B-cell
B) T-cell
C) Null cell
D) All of the above

57. In anaemia of chronic diseases laboratory findings are:
A) Serum iron decreases
B) TIBC decreases
C) Ferritin decreases
D) All of the above

58. Hb Bart's is represented as:
A) Alpha 4
B) Beta 4
C) Gamma 4
D) Delta 4

59. Bernard Soulier syndrome is associated with all except:
A) Large size platelet
B) Reduced platelet count
C) Ristocetin is normal
D) ADP is normal

60. Pancytopaenia with bone marrow hypercellularity is seen in:
A) G6PD deficiency
B) Myelodysplasia
C) PNH
D) Megaloblastic anaemia

61. Patient with haemophilia is characterized by all except:
A) Male
B) Haemarthrosis
C) Purpura
D) Echymosis

62. All causes pancytopaenia except:
A) Cerebellar haemangioblastoma
B) Hypernephroma
C) Pancreatic carcinoma
D) Hepatoma

63. DIC is present in:
A) Hodgkin's lymphoma
B) AML A3
C) CML
D) ALL

64. All of the following are true for promyelocytic leukaemia except:
A) Associated with DIC
B) Translocation 15:17
C) Retinoids are used in treatment
D) CD marker 15 and 34 positive

65. Dense bodies in platelet contains:
A) Serotonin
B) Nucleotides
C) Calcium
D) All of the above

66. Which of the following component is deficient in grey platelet syndrome?
A) Alpha granules
B) Canalicular system
C) Dense bodies
D) Lysosomes

67. Which of the coagulation factor is deficient in haemophilia C.
A) Factor VIII
B) Factor IX
C) Factor XI
D) Factor X

68. Macrocytic anaemia is found in all of the following except:
A) Hypothyroidism
B) Crohn's disease
C) Chronic alcoholism
D) Chronic uraemia

69. Which of the following investigation least useful in multiple myeloma:
A) Urine protein
B) Bone marrow biopsy
C) X-ray
D) Bone scan

70. All of the following is present in warm type of autoimmune haemolytic anaemia except:
A) Jaundice

B) Splenomegaly
C) Raynaud's phenomenon
D) Positive direct Coombs' test

71. All of the following can occur with incompatible blood transfusion except:
A) Fever, rigors
B) Hypotension
C) Bilirubinuria
D) Haemoglobinuria

72. Megaloblastic anaemia is caused by:
A) Vitamin B_6 deficiency
B) Sickle cell anaemia
C) Hereditary orotic aciduria
D) Renal failure

73. von-Willebrand factor is present in:
A) Azurophil granules
B) Specific granule
C) Delta granules
D) Alpha granules

74. Alpha granules are present in:
A) Neutrophils
B) Eosinophil
C) Platelet
D) Mast cell

75. All of the following are complications of thalassaemia except:
A) Haemosiderosis
B) Hepatitis C virus infection
C) Paraproteinaemia
D) HCC

76. Which factor decline fastest in stored blood.
A) Factor V
B) Fibrinogen
C) Fibronectin
D) Prothrombin

77. Disseminated intravascular coagulation is common in:
A) Amniotic fluid embolism
B) Air embolism
C) Fat embolism
D) Thromboembolism

78. Normal life span of eosinophil
A) 1 day
B) 4 days
C) 10 days
D) 20 days

79. Reilly bodies are most commonly seen in which disorder?
A) Acute lymphocytic leukaemia
B) Chronic lymphocytic leukaemia
C) Hodgkin's lymphoma
D) Alder's syndrome

80. CD20 positive cells are:
A) T lymphocytes
B) B lymphocytes
C) Both
D) None

81. What are Faggot cells
A) Myeloblast with azurophilic granules
B) Cells with hypercondensed chromatin
C) Cell that exhibit nuclear cytoplasm asynchrony
D) Cell with multiple Auer rods occurring in bundles

82. Which of the following is/are observed in the peripheral smear after splenectomy?
A) Heinz bodies
B) Pappenheimer bodies
C) Cabot ring
D) Howell Jolly bodies

83. Which of the cells contain peroxidase granules.
A) Basophil
B) Eosinophil
C) Both
D) None

84. Which of the following is found in the secondary granules of neutrophils.
A) Lipase
B) Myeloperoxidase
C) B_{12} binding protein
D) Nucleotidase

85. Excessive reticulocytes are seen in peripheral smear in except:
A) Microangiopathic anaemia
B) Vitamin B_{12} therapy

C) Aplastic anaemia
D) Iron therapy

86. Well-diffentiated lymphocytic lymphoma may involve peripheral blood in?
A) Less than 10%
B) Up to 40%
C) Up to 50%
D) More than 50%

87. Cabot ring is not seen in:
A) Lead poisoning
B) Pernicious anaemia
C) Haemolytic anaemia
D) Iron deficiency anaemia

88. Which of the following causes monocytosis?
A) Typhoid fever
B) Parasitic infections
C) Acute haemorrhage
D) CLL

89. Size of megakaryocyte is:
A) 10 μm
B) 30 μm
C) 40 μm
D) 90 μm

90. Cause of monocytic leukaemoid reaction is
A) Tuberculosis
B) Leishmaniasis
C) Lysosomal storage diseases
D) All of the above

91. Smudge cells are seen in:
A) Burkitt's lymphoma
B) Chronic lymphatic leukaemia
C) Infectious mononucleosis
D) Sezary syndrome

92. Plasma cell are seen in peripheral smear in:
A) Rubella
B) Multiple myeloma
C) Plasma cell leukaemia
D) All of the above

93. Large number of schistocytes are seen in.
A) Microangiopathic haemolytic anaemia
B) Megaloblastic anaemia
C) Vitamin B_6 anaemia
D) Iron deficiency anaemia

94. Which of the following is not a characteristics of multiple myeloma:
A) Increased plasma cells in the BM
B) Osteolytic lesions in bones
C) Increased levels of normal immnunoglobulins
D) Light chains are excreted in urine

95. Atypical lymphocytes are seen in peripheral smear in:
A) Acute lymphatic leukaemia
B) Chronic lymphatic leukaemia
C) Hodgkin's lymphoma
D) Infectious mononucleosis

96. Platelet transfusion is indicated in:
A) Immune thrombocytopaenic purpura
B) Thrombotic thrombocytopaenic purpura
C) Leukaemia
D) Disseminated intravascular coagulation

97. Normal life span of platelet is:
A) 3 days
B) 5days
C) 8 days
D) 20 days

98. Following are the indications of giving cryoprecipitate except:
A) Vitamin K deficiency
B) Haemophilia
C) Hypofibrinogenaemia
D) Disseminated intravascular coagulation

99. Burr cells are seen in **peripheral smear:**
A) Anaemia
B) Renal failure
C) Lead poisoning
D) Leukaemia

100. Basophilic stippling is seen in smear except:
A) Myelophthisic process
B) Myelofibrosis
C) Lead poisoning
D) Iron deficiency anaemia

101. Growth stimulants and inhibitors are produced by:
A) Eosinophils
B) RBCs

C) Macrophages
D) Platelets

102. Congenital disorders of platelet functions are except:
A) Bernard-Soulier syndrome
B) von-Willebrand disease
C) Glanzmann thrombasthenia
D) Storage pool disease

103. von-Willebrand disease is severe in:
A) Blood group AB
B) Blood group O
C) Blood group A
D) Blood group B

104. Prothrombin time is prolonged in:
A) von-Willebrand disease
B) Haemophilia
C) Disseminated intravascular coagulation
D) Uraemia

105. Prothrombin time is prolonged in following conditions except:
A) Vitamin K deficiency
B) Factor V deficiency
C) Glanzmann's thrombasthenia
D) Disseminated intravascular coagulation

106. Amyloid purpura is due to deficiency of factor:
A) Factor V
B) Factor VIII
C) Factor IX
D) Factor X

107. Following are absolute indications of bone marrow biopsy except:
A) Megaloblastic anaemia
B) Multiple myeloma
C) Chronic myeloid leukaemia
D) Idiopathic thrombocytopaenic purpura

108. Immediate response of tissue injury is :
A) Neutropaenia
B) Neutrophilia
C) Monocytosis
D) Eosinophilia

109. Time taken for acute graft-versus host disease after post transfusion is:
A) Before 100 days
B) After 100 days
C) After 150 days
D) After 200 days

110. Graft versus host disease is:
A) Immunologic phenomenon
B) Seen in immunocompromized patients
C) Patient is not histoincompatible
D) None of the above

111. The classic triad of Hand-Schuller-Christian disease includes lesions of bone, exophthalamos and
A) Diabetes mellitus
B) Hepatosplenomegaly
C) Diabetes insipidus
D) Albuminuria

112. In Chediak-Higashi syndrome circulating leukocytes under normal condition demonstrate:
A) Pavementing
B) Margination
C) Giant granules
D) Chemotaxis

113. Excess alpha clumps in erythrocytes in thalassaemia precipitate as insoluble inclusion called as:
A) Howell-Jolly bodies
B) Fessas bodies
C) Rushton bodies
D) Russel bodies

114. Hair-on-end appearance in skull radiograph is seen in:
A) Thalassaemia
B) Sickle cell anaemia
C) Central haemangioma
D) All of the above

115. In heterozygous sickle cell trait is observed when there is a significant:
A) Iron deficiency
B) Hepatosplenomegaly

C) Hypoxia
D) Stasis

116. Hairy cell leukaemia is due to proliferation of:
A) T cells
B) B cells
C) Myeloid cells
D) Macrophages

117. Howell –Jolly bodies are seen after:
A) Hepatectomy
B) Splenectomy
C) Pancreactomy
D) Cholecystectomy

118. Which is not a feature of HELLP syndrome?
A) Haemolytic anaemia
B) Thrombocytopaenia
C) Eosinophilia
D) Raised liver enzyme

119. FIGLU excretion in the urine is an index of the deficiency of:
A) Thiamine
B) Niacin
C) Pyridoxine
D) Folate

120. Transfusion of one unit factor VIII concentrate will raise the level by:
A) 1%
B) 2%
C) 10%
D) 25%

121. All of the following are true about idiopathic thrombocytopaenic purpura except:
A) Megakaryocytes are increased in marrow
B) Chronic form more common in females
C) Patients usually have splenomegaly
D) Splenectomy cures most of them

122. One gm of haemoglobin liberates— mg of bilirubin.
A) 40
B) 10
C) 34
D) 55

123. Microcytic hypochromic anaemia is seen in A/E
A) Lead poisoning
B) Thalassaemia minor
C) Iron deficiency
D) Fanconi's anaemia

124. Which of the following is NOT seen in sickle cells anaemia:
A) Leucopaenia
B) Pulmonary hypertension
C) Fish mouth vertebra
D) Splenic infarct

125. Platelet transfusion is not indicated in:
A) Diluted thrombocytopaenia
B) Immunogenic thrombocytopaenia
C) Aplastic anaemia
D) Leukaemia

126. Thrombocytopaenia is not seen in
A) HS purpura
B) DIC
C) Leukaemia
D) Myelonephrosis

127. All are seen in haemolytic anaemia Except:
A) Haemosiderinuria
B) Reticulocytosis
C) Spherocytosis
D) Increased haptoglobulin

128. Incorrect in pernicious anaemia:
A) Autoimmune disease
B) Hyperchlorhydria
C) Premature graying of hair
D) Parenteral vit B_{12}

129. DIC is seen in all/EXCEPT
A) Diabetes mellitus
B) Amniotic fluid embolism
C) Accidental haemorrhage
D) PPH

130. Predominant in CLL
A) T lymphocytes
B) B-lymphocytes
C) K-cells
D) Helper T cells

131. Hand- Schuller Christian disease which is correct:
A) Proliferation of RE cells
B) Foam cells seen
C) Punched out lesions in X-ray
D) All of the above

132. Bone marrow biopsy is useful in the diagnosis of:
A) CML
B) ALL
C) Aleukaemic leukaemia
D) Hodgkin's lymphoma

133. Confirmation of myelofibrosis is by:
A) Bone marrow aspiration
B) Bone marrow biopsy
C) Peripheral smear
D) Splenic puncture

134. Chloroma is a tumour of:
A) Soft tissue
B) Bone
C) Haemopietic tissue
D) Ovary

135. Repeated blood transfusion can cause all of the following except:
A) Haemosiderosis
B) Pulmonary edema
C) Thrombocytopaenia
D) Thromboembolism

136. Preservative used for storage of blood for transfusion is:
A) Heparin + glucose
B) Citrate +glucose
C) EDTA
D) CPD—A

137. Factor deficiency in Christmas disease is:
A) II
B) VII
C) VIII
D) IX

138. Massive blood transfusion is defined as:
A) 350 ml in 5 minutes
B) 500 ml in 5 minutes
C) 1 litre in 5 minutes
D) Whole blood volume

139. Glycosylated haemoglobin assay is helpful in the monitoring of patients in:
A) Addison's disease
B) Diabetes mellitus
C) Cushing's syndrome
D) Grave's disease

140. In acute loss of blood the cellular compensation is reflected by release of:
A) RBCs
B) Platelets
C) Reticulocytes
D) Haemosiderin

141. Nuclear cytoplasmic asynchrony is characteristic feature of:
A) Megaloblastic anaemia
B) Iron deficiency anaemia
C) Erythroblastosis fetalis
D) All of the above

142. Congenital aplastic anaemia associated with syndrome is called:
A) Cooley's anaemia
B) Sickle cell anaemia
C) Gray baby syndrome
D) Fanconi's anaemia

143. Pathogenesis of thalassaemia is:
A) Reduced in haemoglobin concentration
B) Defect in haemoglobin synthesis
C) Decrease in RBC count
D) All of the above

144. Paul Bunnell test is positive in:
A) Cyclic neutropaenia
B) Agranulocytosis
C) Leukaemia
D) Infectious mononucleosis

145. Deficiency of all the three components of coagulation factor VIII result in:
A) von-Willebrand disease
B) Haemophilia A
C) Parahaemophilia
D) Haemophilia B

Answers

1. A) Heinz bodies are single or multiple, round to oval globules 1-2 μ in diameter. They are eosinophilic with Romanosky's stain. They are readily demonstrated in supraviolet methyl violet preparation or stained by brilliant cresyl blue. They are also seen in phase contrast and dark background microscopy. They represent aggregates of denatured haemoglobin. They are seen in G6PD deficiency, chemically induced anaemia and after splenectomy.

2. C) Coombs' test discovered by Coombs' for detecting non-agglutinating (incomplete) blood group antibodies in serum and also complement components attached to red cells. Indications of direct Coombs' test include haemolytic transfusion reaction, diagnosis of haemolytic disease of newborn, detection of cold and warm antibodies, and autoimmune drug induced haemolytic anaemia.

3. C) pH of tris EDTA boric acid buffer is 8.6.

4. A) Investigations suggests intravascular haemolysis are as follows:

(a) Serum haptoglobin reduced
(b) Plasma methemalbumin present
(c) Haemoglobinuria
(d) Haemosiderinuria
(e) Increased plasma haemoglobin

5. C) Normal amount A2 haemoglobin in RBCs is 3% In α thalassaemia minor or heterozygous α thalasaemia there is increased in haemoglobin A2 (5%).

6. A) Bence-Jones protein is a monoclonal globulin protein found in the blood or urine with a molecular weight 22 kD a. Bence-Jones protein is present in urine in cases of multiple myeloma, Waldenstrom's macroglobulinaemia, chronic lymphatic leukaemia, amyloidosis, lymphomas, osteogenic sarcoma, cryoglobulinaemia, malignant B cell disease and metastatic carcinoma.

7. C) Structure of HBH is β_4. Haemoglobin H is β chain tetramers. It is present in cases of homozygous alpha thalassaemia in adults. Patient with Hb H disease presents with haemolytic anaemia, splenomegaly and cholelithiasis. γ_4 is haemoglobin Bart present in homozygous alpha thalassaemia in infants. $\alpha_2 \beta_2$ is adult haemoglobin and $\alpha_2 \gamma_2$ is haemoglobin F.

8. C) Coagulation disorders include Christmas disease, von-Willebrand disease, disseminated intravascular coagulation and certain drugs.

9. B) Howell Jolly bodies are purple black usually round chromatic fragments. They are usually single and are larger and more deeply stained than the granules of basophilic stippling. Howell Jolly bodies are seen in disorder such as megaloblastic anaemia, but appear in red cells after splenectomy.

10. A) Hyposegmented neutrophils are seen in chronic myeloid leukaemia.

11. B) Structure of Hb F is $\alpha_2 \gamma_2$.

12. B) About 25% of total iron content is an intracellular storage pool composed of iron storage proteins haemosiderin and ferritin. Ferritin contains 23% of ferric iron gives Prussian blue reaction stained light blue coloured small granules. It is colourless in tissues. Equally distributed in reticuloendothelial system, hepatocytes and skeletal muscle cells. Ferritin is less stable, readily available for haemoglobin synthesis. Ferritin has an outer shell of non-iron apoferritin-protein shell. It is trivalent iron-central core of molecular weight of apoferritin is 45000.

13. B) It is estimated that 20% to 60% of those having cerebral infarction will have second attack. The etiology of cerebral occlusion in sickle cell anemia is that sickling of red cells is thought to be initiated by hypoxaemia. Capillary engorgement with sickle cell leads to coagulation and retrograde thrombosis of small vessels. Stasis in the vasa-vasorum of larger vessels may lead to proliferation of the intima and media with eventual occlusion or the intimal defects may serve as a focus for clot formation within the vessels.

14. B) Myeloma cell varies in size, from 15 to 25µm, the cytoplasm has a deep blue colour, is non-granular and usually shows a pale perinuclear clear area or "hof" representing Golgi zone. The nucleus is generally eccentric but may be situated centrally within the cytoplasm but lacks the cartwheel appearance. The nuclear chromatin appears to be in the form of a loose mesh; several nucleoli may be discernable and are usually more obvious in the myeloma cells. Russell bodies consisting of hyaline globules of immunoglobulin are present in the cytoplasm. Binucleated or multinucleated plasma cells are present. Intracellular accumulations of immunoglobulins may produce distinctive morphological features such as Mott cells or Morula cells (numerous 'grape like' pale bluish cytoplasmic inclusions).

15. B) Causes of neutropaenia include typhoid, tuberculosis, influenza, dengue, measles, megaloblastic anaemia, malaria, kala-azar, aplastic anaemia, drug induced bone marrow depression, radiation, myelofibrosis and hypersplenism. Rhinovirus is a causative organism of common cold does not cause leukopaenia.

16. C) On haemoglobin electrophoresis fastest moving abnormal haemoglobin is HbH.

17. B) Henoch-Schonlein purpura (HSP) or anaphylactoid purpura is an immunoglobulin (IgA) mediated small blood vessel vasculitis that predominantly affects children but also is seen in adults. HSP is a subset of necrotizing vasculitis characterized by fibrinoid destruction of blood vessels and leukocytosis. Clinical presentations include, palpable purpura, arthralgia, or arthritis, abdominal pain, and gastrointestinal bleeding.

18. A) Haemoglobins which crosses hemoglobin A band on cellulose acetate strips are hemoglobin J, Hb H, Hb Bart, Hb K, Hb I. Band of Hb D is present before the band of Hb A.

19. C) Hypersegmented neutrophils are seen in pernicious anaemia.

20. C) Philadelphia chromosome or Philadelphia translocation is a specific chromosomal abnormality that is associated with chronic myeloid leukaemia, It is the result of a reciprocal translocation between chromosome 9 and 22 and is specially designed (9-22) (q34:q11) is seen. However Philadelphia (Ph) chromosome is not sufficiently specific to diagnose CML, since it is found in acute lymphoblastic leukaemia.

21. C) Anaemia of chronic disease is increasingly referred to anaemia of inflammation is a form of anaemia seen in chronic illness. Causes of anaemia of chronic diseases are as follows:

1. Inflammatory conditions: Tuberculosis, syphilis, lung abscess, endocarditis
2. Collagen disorders: Rheumatoid arthritis, systemic lupus erythematosus, ulcerative colitis, Crohn's disease
3. Metabolic: Uremia (renal failure)
4. Malignancy: Hodgkin's lymphoma, lung cancer and breast cancer.

22. D) Cytogenitic translocations associated with specific genetic abnormalities in acute lymphatic leukaemia are t (9:22), t (8-14). t (15;17) is associated consistently with AML-M3.

23. D) Microcytic hypochromic anaemia includes, iron deficiency anaemia, sideroblastic anaemia, thalassaemia, and anaemia of chronic disorder, vitamin B_6 deficiency and hereditary spherocytosis. Vitamin C deficiency causes macrocytic hypochromic anaemia.

24. B) In folic acid deficiency type of anaemia is macrocytic hypochromic. Sickle cell anaemia causes normocytic normochromic anaemia and in cases of myelofibrosis there is aplastic anaemia.

25. C) Vitamin B_6 causes microcytic hypochromic anaemia, Macrocytic hypochromic anaemia is caused by folic acid deficiency, vitamin B_{12} deficiency, liver diseases, hypothyroidism, alcoholism and vitamin C deficiency.

26. B) Anaemia of chronic infection is characterized by microcytic hypochromic anaemia, decreased TIBC, increased serum ferritin and decreased MCHC.

27. A) MCHC is increased in spherocytosis. Normal MCHC is 32-36%. It is decreased in hypochromic anaemia, macrocytic anaemia.

28. C) Normal myeloid erythroid ratio is 3:1.

29. D) Diseases transmitted by blood transfusion included, AIDS, hepatitis B, hepatitis C, syphilis, malaria, leishmaniasis, cytomegalovirus, brucellosis, and toxoplasma gondii infection.

30. C) Size of filter used in blood transfusion set is 170 micrometer.

31. B) Cryoprecipitate is called "cryoprecipitated antihaemophilic factor" is a frozen blood product prepared from plasma. Cryoprecipitate contains, factor VIII. fibrinogen, von-Willebrand factor, factor XIII and fibrinonectin. Anti-thrombin is not present in cryoprecipitate.

32. B) Bone marrow iron is increased when there is iron overload, in infections, dyserythropoietic anaemias, sideroblastic anaemia, and thalassaemia. Decreased or absent bone marrow iron is seen in granulocytic leukaemia, polycythaemia and iron deficiency anaemia. Individuals with polycythaemia vera use iron very rapidly to produce the increased cell mass.

33. C) In abnormal red cell disorders such as poikilocytosis, spherocytosis and sickle cell anaemia there is no rouleaux formation. ESR is very slow. ESR is slow in polycythaemia, congestive cardiac failure and hypofibrinogenaemia.

ESR is increased in:

1. Chronic infection: Tuberculosis, chronic osteomyelitis, chronic bronchiectasis, chronic lung abscess.
2. Autoimmune diseases: SLE, rheumatoid arthritis, acute rheumatic fever.
3. Acute inflammation: Acute myocardial infarction, any extensive inflammation.
4. Neoplasms: Hodgkin's lymphoma, leukaemia, carcinomatosis, multiple myeloma.

34. C) Normal mean corpuscular volume is 90 femtoliter.

35. B) One unit of fresh blood rises the Hb % concentration by 1 gram.

36. B) Blood is stored at +2° to +6° C.

37. C) Chronic myeloid leukaemia is characterized by anaemia, decreased neutrophilic alkaline phosphatase, increased WBCs count and thrombocytosis.

38. D) Recurrent cytogenetic abnormalities are strong prognostic indicators in AML.

39. B) Sickle cell anaemia is associated with infarction of bones, brain, spleen and kidney. There is hepatosplenomegaly, leg ulcers, osteomyelitis, and pneumonia and retinal vessel obstruction. In males, in sickle cell anaemia there is improper development of gonads and secondary sex characters priapism a painful persistent erection of penis often occurs, this is because of vascular stasis and accentuated sickling within corpora cavernosa. In females during pregnancy intrauterine growth retardation and increased fetal wastage is done.

40. D) Hazards of exchange transfusions are hypocalcaemia, citrate toxicity, hyperkalemia, perforation of vessels, thrombosis, infarction, arrhythmias, thrombocyto-paenia (bleeding, infections, haemolysis, and graft-versus-host disease).

41. A) Commonest cause of aplastic anaemia is idiopathic.

42. B) In the normal 120-day life span of the red blood cell, glucose molecules react with haemoglobin, forming glycated. In individuals with poorly controlled diabetes, the quantities of these glycated haemoglobins are much higher than in healthy people. In general, the reference range is about 4% to 5.7%. High levels of $HbA1_C$ are found in people with persistently elevated blood sugar, as in diabetes mellitus.

43. C) Bloom syndrome also known as Bloom-Torre-Machacek syndrome is a rare autosomal recessive chromosomal disorder characterized by a high frequency of breaks and rearrangements in an affected person's chromosomes. Dermatologist Dr David Bloom in 1954 discovered the condition. The greatly elevated rate of mutation in Bloom syndrome results in a high risk of cancer in affected individuals. Patients are predisposed to leukaemias, lymphoma and. Fanconi's anaemia is a genetic disease that affects children and adults from all ethnic backgrounds. Many patients eventually develop acute myelogenous leukaemia, oesophageal, gastrointestinal and vulvar carcinoma. Patau syndrome is associated with malignancy. AIDS is an acquired disease not a genetic disorder.

44. D) Haemoglobinopathies include thalassaemia, sickle cell anaemia, Hb E, D, I, J, k, Hb Bart and Hb H disease.

45. A) Commonest cause of anaemia in childhood is iron deficiency anaemia.

46. C) For acute leukaemia the blast cells should be more than 30%

47. D) Thalassaemia major is characterized by microcytic hypochromic anaemia, increased HbF and target cell are present in peripheral blood. Osmotic fragility is decreased.

48. C) Acute myeloid leukaemia occurs in adults and old age. Promyelocytic leukaemia is a disease of childhood. Cases are reported 2-17 years of age. In this case patient is young with thrombocytopaenia leading to bleeding from gum and eye.

49. C) One unit platelet increases platelet count by 5000 platelets per cmm. Patient received 8 units of platelets. Therefore total number of platelets transfused is 40,000 platelets cmm. Patient's platelet count was 75000 cmm. Post-transfusion platelet will be 115000 cu mm.

50. C) Hereditary spherocytosis is an autosomal dominant or recessive trait. It is caused by a variety of molecular defects in the genes that code for spectrin, ankyrin, band-3 protein, protein 4.2 and anion exchanger transporter deficiency.

51. B) In acute promyelocytic leukaemia translocation is seen in chromosome (15-17).

52. C) Heterozygous thalassaemia presents as microcytic hypochromic anaemia. Smear shows target cells. Clinically symptomless. There is increased haemoglobin A_2 (5%).

53. A) Autoimmune haemolytic anaemia is associated with B cell lymphoma.

54. C) In a patient with thalassaemia peripheral smear shows features of microcytic hypochromic anaemia.

55. D) Causes of microangiopathic haemolytic anaemia include haemolytic uraemic syndrome, disseminated intravascular coagulation, thrombotic thrombocytopaenic purpura, malignant hypertension, paraneoplastic syndrome, mitomycin C and Schulman Upshaw syndrome.

56. C) Commonest type of ALL is Null cell (85%) and has good prognosis. There are major subgroups of acute lymphoblastic leukaemia. They are T-cell, B-cell and Null cell. B-cell leukaemias are (2%). T-cell leukaemia forms 10% of ALL and has poor prognosis.

57. D) In chronic diseases, serum iron decreases, TIBC decreases, ferritin decreases, and MCHC decreases.

58. C) Haemoglobin Bart's is represented as Gamma 4. γ_4 is haemogobin Bart present in homozygous alpha thalassaemia in infants.

59. C) Laboratory findings in Bernard Soulier syndrome are:

1. Bleeding time is markedly prolonged.
2. Platelet count is variable. There is mild to moderate thrombocytopaenia.
3. Peripheral blood smear shows macroplatelets (>3.5 to 20μm).
4. Bone marrow: Megakaryocytes, normal or increased.
5. Platelet aggregation in the presence of ristocin and botrocetin decreased or absent and not corrected by addition of normal plasma.
6. Platelet aggregation induced by agonists such as ADP, collagen, thrombin and epinephrine is normal.

60. D) In megaloblastic anemia there is leukopaenia, anaemia and thrombocytopaenia with hypercellularity of bone marrow. In G6PD deficiency there is anaemia with hypercellular bone marrow. Leukocyte and platelet count is normal. In cases of PNH and myelodysplasia bone marrow is hypocellular with pancytopaenia.

61. C) Haemophilia is characterized by haemarthroses, haematomas, haematuria, haemorrhage into the central nervous system, mucus membrane haemorrhage, pseudotumours, dental and surgical bleeding.

62. C) Pancytopaenia is caused by cerebellar haemangioblastoma, hypernephroma, hepatoma, testicular sarcoma, melanoma, bronchogenic carcinoma, metastatic carcinoma breast and lung.

63. B) Intravascular disseminated coagulation is associated with acute promyelocytic leukaemia.

64. D) Acute promyelocytic leukaemia is a subtype of acute myelogenous leukaemia (AML) a cancer of blood and bone marrow. It is also known as progranulocytic leukaemia (APL); AML with t (15:17) (q22:q12). The disease is characterized by a chromosomal translocation involving retinoic acid receptor alpha gene and is unique from other form of AML, in its responsiveness to all transretinoic acid (ATRA) therapy. It is frequently associated with bleeding caused by disseminated intravascular coagulation (DIC). Expression of CD15 is a marker of cellular differentiation in cervical intraepithelial neoplasia. CD34 is a useful marker in determining tumour neovascularization, which might be of prognostic relevance in patients with ovarian tumours.

65. D) Dense bodies of platelets contain serotonin, nucleotides, calcium, and lysosomes containing hydrolytic enzyme.

66. A) Grey platelet syndrome or platelet alpha-granule deficiency is a rare congenital bleeding disorder caused by a reduction or absence of the platelets, or of the proteins contained in these granules. It is generally inherited as an autosomal dominant manner, although a few recessive cases have been noted.

67. C) Haemophilia C is a mild form of haemophilia affecting both sexes. It is caused by a deficiency of coagulation factor XI and is distinguished from haemophilia A and B by the fact that it does not lead to bleeding into the joints. Haemophilia A is caused by factor VIII deficiency and haemophilia B is caused by factor X deficiency.

68. D) In chronic uraemia or chronic renal failure there is microcytic hypochromic anaemia. Causes of macrocytic hypochromic anaemia include vitamin B_{12} deficiency, folic acid deficiency, hypothyroidism, antiepileptic medication, liver disease, Crohn's disease and chronic alcoholism.

69. D) Bence-Jones protein is a monoclonal globulin protein found in the blood or urine with a molecular weight 22 kD a. Bence-Jones protein is present in urine in cases of multiple myeloma. Malignant plasma cells are present in parts of the bone marrow involved. They may form clumps or sheets, which replace the marrow, or may be scattered among the normal haemopoietic cells. X-ray skull shows small well-circumscribed areas of rarefaction of bone. Classically lesions are seen as punched out defects in the bone.

70. C) Warm antibody autoimmune haemolytic anaemia is characterized by anaemia, jaundice, splenomegaly and positive direct Coombs' test. Uneven bluish or reddish discolouration of the skin of the digits, ankles, and wrist (acrocynosis or Raynaud's sign) is a feature of cold autoimmne haemolytic anaemia.

71. C) There is no bilirubinuria though the bilirubin is increased in blood. Complications of mismatched blood transfusion include fever with rigor, jaundice, hypotension, back pain, chest pain, dyspnea, tachycardia, rashes, haemoglobinuria, haemosiderinuria, and decreased haptoglobin in serum.

72. C) Megaloblastic anaemia is caused by hereditary orotic aciduria. Orotic aciduria refers to an excessive excretion of orotic acid in urine. Its hereditary form, an autosomal recessive disorder can be caused by deficiency of enzyme UMPS. Patients cannot be cured by administration of vitamin B_{12} or folic acid. It can cause inhibition of RNA or DNA.

73. D) von-Willebrand factor is present in alpha granules of platelets.

74. C) Alpha granules are present in platelets. Alpha granules of platelet contain platelet factor 4, transforming growth factor-B_1, platelet derived growth factor, B-thromboglobulin, fibronectin, vWF, fibrinogen, coagulation factor V and XIII.

75. C) Beta thalassaemia is the most common haemoglobinopathy with treatment of regular blood transfusion. Iron overload and haemosiderosis can involve heart, kidney, pancreas, liver and lung. Due to repeated blood transfusion hepatitis B, C and HIV infection occur. Hepatocellular carcinoma is a complication of cirrhosis. Due to repeated blood transfusion, patients with beta thalassaemia are often infected with either hepatitis C or hepatitis B virus. Hepatocellular carcinoma frequently complicates hepatic cirrhosis secondary to viral infection.

76. A) Factor V activity falls to 50% after 14 days of preservation.

77. A) Disseminated intravascular coagulation is common with amniotic fluid embolism. During parturition amniotic fluid enter a uterine vein, especially after manipulations. The cause of amniotic fluid embolism include rupture of amniotic sac, ruptured uterine and cervical veins and pressure gradient from uterus to vein. Other obstetric complications causing disseminated intravascular coagulation are placental abruption, various types of abortions, retained dead fetus, pregnancy induced hypertension molar pregnancy.

78. C) Normal life span of eosinophils is 8-12 days.

79. D) Reilly bodies are seen in Alder's syndrome. Alder's-Reilly anomaly is associated with the genetic mucopolysaccharidoses lack the lysosomal enzymes necessary to break down polysaccharides. Dense azurophilic granules, resembling toxic granulation in neutrophils are seen in all leukocytes. Most characteristic of these disorders is metachromatic granules surrounded by a clear zone seen in lymphocytes.

80. B) CD20 is a non-glycosylated phosphoprotein expressed on the surface of mature B-cell lymphocytes

81. D) Faggot cell is a term used for cells normally found in the hypergranular form of acute promyelocytic leukaemia (FAB-3). The term is applied to those blast cells because of numerous Auer rods in the cytoplasm. The accumulation of these Auer rods gives the bundles of sticks, from which the cells are given their names.

82. D) Heinz bodies are seen in G6PD deficiency and drug induced haemolytic anaemia. Cabot rings are observed in megaloblastic anaemia and lead poisoning. Howell Jolly bodies are seen in splenectomy patients. Pappenheimer bodies are seen in macrocytic anaemia.

83. C) Granules of basophils and eosinophils contain peroxidase enzyme.

84. C) Secondary granules of neutrophils contain lysozymes, lactoferrin, collagenase and cationic protein.

85. C) Causes of reticulocytosis include haemolytic anaemia, response to vitalmin B_{12} therapy, response to iron therapy and bone marrow stimulation. It is decreased in aplastic anaemia

86. A) Well-differentiated lymphocytic lymphoma (small cell lymphocytic lymphoma) may involve peripheral blood in less than 10% of cases.

87. D) Cabot ring appears as red purple round or figure of eight structure with Leishman stain. It is seen in peripheral smear in cases of lead poisoning, pernicious anaemia, haemolytic anaemia and leukaemia.

88. A) Monocytosis is seen in typhoid fever. In parasitic infestation there is eosinophilia. There is neutrophilia in acute haemorrhage and CLL shows lymphocytosis.

Causes of monocytosis

Chronic infections

Bacterial: Subacute bacterial endocarditis, tuberculosis, brucellosis, typhoid fever

Protozoal: Malaria, leishmaniasis, trypanosomiasis

Rickettsial: Typus, Rocky mountain spotted fever

Malignancy: Hodgkin's lymphoma, carcinomatosis

Haematological: Chronic myelomonocytic leukaemia, acute monocytic leukaemia, myeloproliferative disorders.

Marrow recovery after cytotoxic therapy

Lipoid storage diseases

89. D) Normal size of megakaryocyte varies from 50 μm to 100 μm.

90. D) Causes of monocytic leukaemoid reaction include, tuberculosis, lysosomal storage disorders, and leishmaniasis.

91. B) Smudge cells or basket cells are leukocytes that have damaged during preparation of the peripheral blood smear. This usually occurs due to the fragility of the cell. They are usually seen in chronic lymphocytic leukaemia.

92. D) Plasma cells are normally not seen in peripheral smear. They are present in smear in rubella, multiple myeloma, and plasma cell leukaemia.

93. A) Schistocytes are variously sized and shaped fragments of red blood cells. They are seldom present in normal blood. When present in large number in peripheral blood, a haemolytic process is suggested.

Causes of schistocytosis are: Microangiopathic haemolytic anaemia, disseminated intravascular coagulation, haemolytic uremic syndrome, giant haemangioma, and metastatic carcinoma.

94. C) In cases of multiple myeloma there is increase in M protein in the serum. There is hyperglobulinaemia. Normal immnunoglobulins are decreased. Urine examination shows presence of Bence-Jones protein. X-ray skull shows small well-demarcated areas of rarefaction of bone. There are increased plasma cells in bone marrow.

95. D) Atypical lymphocytes are lymphocytes with abundant finely granular, basophilic cytoplasm containing small fenestrations.

96. C) Platelet transfusions are traditionally given to those underlying chemotherapy for leukaemia, aplastic anaemia, thrombocytopaenia, AIDS, hypersplenism, sepsis, bone marrow transplant, radiation treatment, organ transplant or surgeries such as cardiopulmonary bypass.

Platelet transfusions should be avoided in those with thrombotic thrombocytopaenic purpura (TTP) because it can worsen neurological symptoms and acute renal failure presumably due to a creation of new thrombi as platelets are consumed. It should be avoided in those with heparin-induced thrombocytopaenia or disseminated intravascular coagulation (DIC). Patients with immune thrombocytopaenia, include idiopathic thrombocytopaenic purpura or drug induced thrombocytopaenia. Platelet transfusion is not recommended for this group of patients because the underlying cause involves antibodies that destroy platelets, therefore any newly transfused platelets will also be destroyed.

97. C) Normal life span of platelets is 8-10 days. Life span of transfused platelets is 2-3 days.

98. A) Cryoprecipitate contains factor VIII, fibrinogen, von-Willebrand factor, and factor XIII. Absolute indication of cryoprecipitate transfusion is in cases of hypofibrinogenaemia. It can be used in cases of von-Willebrand disease, haemophilia and disseminated intravascular coagulation if specific factor is not available.

99. B) Burr cells or helmet cells are normal sized RBCs with one or more long (may be 3.5μm) blunt projections. They are seen in renal failure.

100. D) Basophilic stippling: Small discrete dots in basophilic stippling occur in red blood cell cytoplasm in many haemopoietic disorders such as lead poisoning, aplastic anaemia, thalassaemia, myelodysplasia, and megaloblastosis.

101. D) Platelets release a multitude of growth factors including platelet-derived factor (PDGF), a potent chemotactic agent, and TGF beta, which stimulate the deposition of extracellular matrix. Both of these growth factors have been shown to play a significant role in the repair and regeneration of connective tissues.

Other healing-associated growth factors produced by platelets, include basic fibroblast growth factor, insulin-like growth factor-1, platelet derived epidermal growth factor, and vascular endothelial growth factor.

102. B) Bernard Soulier syndrome, is a rare autosomal recessive bleeding disorder is due to reduced or abnormal platelet membrane expression of glycoprotein Ib/IX (von-Willebrand receptor).

Glanzmann thrombasthenia results from a qualitative abnormality in glycoprotein IIb/IIIa receptors on the platelet membrane, which are required to bind fibrinogen and vWF, both of which bridge platelets during aggregation.

Under normal circumstances, activated platelets release the contents of platelet granules to reinforce the aggregatory response.

Storage pool disease is defect in release of alpha or dense (delta) platelet granules, or both (alpha-delta storage pool disease).

von-Willebrand syndrome is the most common hereditary coagulation abnormality described in humans, although it can also be acquired as a result of other medical conditions. It arises from a quantitative deficiency of von-Willebrand factor (vWF), a multimeric protein that is acquired for platelet adhesion.

103. B) von-Willebrand disease is more severe or apparent in people with blood group O.

104. C) Prothrombin time is prolonged in disseminated intravascular coagulation.

105. C) Prothrombin time is normal in Glanzmann's thrombasthenia

No.	Condition	Prothrombin time
1.	Vitamin K deficiency or Wafarin	Prolonged
2.	Disseminated intravascular coagulation	Prolonged
3.	von-Willebrand disease	Unaffected
4.	Haemophilia	Unaffected
5.	Aspirin	Unaffected
6.	Thrombocytopaenia	Prolonged
7.	Early liver failure	Prolonged
8.	End stage liver failure	Prolonged
9.	Congenital afibrinogenemia	Prolonged
10.	Factor V deficiency	Prolonged
11.	Uremia	Unaffected
12.	Factor X deficiency as seen in amyloid purpura	Prolonged
13.	Glanzmann's thrombasthenia	Unaffected
14.	Bernard-Soulier syndrome	Unaffected

106. D) Amyloid purpura is a condition marked by bleeding under the skin (purpura) in some individuals with amyloidosis. The precise cause of amyloid purpura is unknown, but several mechanisms are thought to contribute. One may be a decrease in the level of circulating factor X, a clotting factor necessary for coagulation. The proposed mechanism for this decrease factor X is that circulating amyloid fibrils bind and inactivate factor X. Another contributing factor may be enhanced fibrinolysis, the breakdown clots. Subendothelial deposits of amyloid may weaken blood vessels and lead to extravasation of blood. Amyloid deposits in GIT and liver may also play a role in development of amyloid purpura.

107. C) Indications of bone marrow biopsy

Anaemia

1. Hypoplastic and aplastic anaemia
2. Megaloblastic anaemia
3. Sideroblastic anaemia
4. Refractory anaemia

Leukaemia

1. Aleukaemic or subleukaemic leukaemia

Idiopathic thrombocytopaenic purpura

Multiple myeloma

Carcinoma

Collagen diseases.

108. B) Neutrophils increased as a result of tissue injury such as myocardial infarction, burn and after surgery.

109. A) Acute graft versus host disease occurs within 100 days of post transplant.

110. A) Graft-versus-host disease (GVHD) is a common complication of allogenic bone marrow transplantation in which functional immune cells in the transplanted marrow recognize the recipient as foreign and mount an immunologic attack. It can also take place in a blood transfusion under certain circumstances. The recipient is immunocompromized and therefore cannot destroy or inactivate the transplanted cells.

The recipient is immunologically disparate-histoincompatible.

111. C) A more localized variant, primarily referred to as Hand- Schuller-Christian disease, or multifocal eosinophilic granuloma is a childhood disease that consists of the triad of diabetes insipidus, lytic bone lesions and proptosis. It is the result of error of metabolism of cholesterol and its esters.

The age group involved is more than 3 years of age. It is more common in boys than girls 2:1.

112. C) A blood smear shows giant granules in the white blood cells. Giant granules are also found in cells from biopsy of skin, muscle and nerves.

113. B) The thalassaemia major is a homozygous β thlassaemia and is characterized by diminished or absent synthesis of the beta chains. Despite impaired synthesis of the beta chains, synthesis of alpha chains continues at a normal rate.

The imbalance results in precipitation of the excess alpha chains (Fossas bodies) in the erythrocytes and membrane damage to the red cells.

Ruston bodies are linear or curved hyaline bodies presumably of haematogenous origin found in the epithelial lining of odontogenic cysts.

114. D) The skull alterations are due to overactivity of the red marrow in response to anaemia. The marrow hyperplasia widens the diploic space and thins the outer table. There is trabecular destruction with thinning of residual trabeculae. The trabecular pattern within the diploae may sometimes be arranged perpendicular to the curvature of the cranial vault. The alternating opaque, thickened trabeculae and radiolucent marrow hyperplasia produce hair-on-end appearance.

Hair on end appearance on radiograph is seen in:

A) Hereditary spherocytosis
B) Iron deficiency anaemia
C) Neuroblastoma
D) Central haemangioma
E) Enzyme deficiency (G6PD) anaemia
F) Sickle cell anaemia
G) Thalassaemia major
H) Ewing's sarcoma
I) Toxoplasmosis
J) Malaria

115. C) Complications of heterogenous sickle cell trait include increased urinary tract infection in women, gross haematuria, and complications of hyphemia, splenic infarction with altitude hypoxia or exercise.

116. B) It is a rare B cell leukaemia. Hairy cell leukaemia accounts 2-5 in 100 number of cases of leukaemia. Male-female ratio is 6:1 and the median age at diagnosis is 50. Hairy cell leukaemia is associated with other immunological disorders including scleroderma, polymyositis, polyarteritis nodosa, erythematous maculopapules and pyoderma gangrenosum.

Hairy cells are small lymphocytes with normal/kidney shaped,/dumbbell shaped nuclei, scanty blue cytoplasm, and hair like projections of the cytoplasm best seen by phase contrast microscopy. The nucleus can be central or eccentric and it can show evidence of indentation or folding. The cytoplasm is agranular stains moderately to light basophilic, and often has an intensely stained periphery and a prominent perinuclear zone.

117. B) Howell Jolly bodies are purple black usually round chromatic fragments. They are usually single and are larger and more deeply stained than the granules of basophilic stippling. Howell Jolly bodies are seen in disorder such as megaloblastic anaemia, but appear in red cells after splenectomy.

118. C) HELLP is an abbreviation of the main findings:

1. Haemolytic anaemia
2. Elevated liver enzymes
3. Low platelet count

HELLP syndrome is a life threatening obstetric complication usually considered to be a variant of pre-eclamsia. Both conditions usually occur during the later stages of pregnancy, or sometimes after childbirth.

The exact cause of HELLP is not unknown:

1. General activation of the coagulation cascade is considered the main underlying problem.

2. Fibrin forms cross-linked network in the small blood vessels. This leads to microangiopathic haemolytic anaemia: the mesh causes destruction of red blood cells as if they were being forced through a strainer.
3. As the liver appears to be the main site of this process, downstream liver cells suffer ischemia leading to periportal necrosis.

HELLP syndrome leads to a various form of disseminated intravascular coagulation (DIC), leading to paradoxical bleeding.

Disseminated intravascular coagulation is also seen in about 20% of all women with HELLP syndrome and 84% when HELLP is complicated by acute renal failure.

119. D) Formiminoglutamic acid (FIGLU) a degradation product of histidine combines with tetrahydrofolate to form N5 Formaminotetrahydrofolate and glutamate. This reaction cannot occur in severe folate deficiency and hence FIGLU and uroconic acid appear in urine on histidine load. This test is employed to detect and assess folic acid deficiency.

120. B) Transfusion of one unit of factor VIII concentrate will raise the level by 2%.

121. D) **Splenectomy is not generally considered in early phases of ITP, in pregnancy or in children under six.**

Bone marrow examination shows:

1. Magakaryocytes are numerous.
2. Many young megakaryocytes— Single nucleus, scanty or moderate cytoplasm and a few granules.
3. Exceptionally large megakaryocytes— non-lobulated nucleus, vaculated cytoplasm, a few granules.
4. Platelets are few around the megakaryocytes.

Chronic ITP is a disease of young to middle aged females.

122. C) Bilirubin is a tetrapyrrole, 80-90% of which is produced in the reticuloendothelial system by breakdown of haemoglobin from effete erythrocytes. Bilirubin is formed in the RE system as a degradation product of haemoglobin liberated from mature RBCs. (1 gram yields approximately 35 mg bilirubin).

123. D) Fanconi's anaemia is a disease passed through families (inherited) that mainly affects the bone marrow. It results in decreased production of all types of blood cells.

Fanconi's anaemia is due to an abnormal gene that damages cells, which keeps them from repairing damaged DNA.

Persons with Fanconi's anaemia have lower than normal numbers of white blood cells, red blood cells, and platelets.

Not enough white blood cells can lead to infections.

A lack of red blood cells may result in fatigue (anaemia)

A lower than normal platelets may lead to excess bleeding.

124. A) **The high blood cell count is found in most patients with sickle cell anaemia.**

In the spine the thinning of the cortical bones of vertebral centra gives rise to biconcave centra, which has a codfish appearance on the lateral X-ray film.

Pulmonary hypertension, diagnosed by droppler echocardiography, is common in adults with sickle cell disease. It appears to be a complication of chronic haemolysis, is resistant to hydroxyurea therapy, and confers a high risk of death.

125. B) Platelet transfusions are traditionally given to those underlying chemotherapy for leukaemia, aplastic anaemia, thrombocytopaemia, AIDS, hypersplenism, sepsis, bone marrow transplant, radiation treatment, organ transplant or surgeries such as cardiopulmonary bypass.

Platelet transfusions should be avoided in those with thrombotic thrombocytopaenic purpura (TTP) because it can worsen neurological symptoms and acute renal failure presumably due to a creation of new thrombi as platelets are consumed. It should be avoided in those with heparin-induced thrombocytopaenia or disseminated intravascular coagulation (DIC). Patients with immune thrombocytopaenia, include idiopathic thrombocytopaenic purpura or drug induced thrombocytopaenia. Platelet transfusion is not recommended for this group of patients because the underlying cause involves antibodies that destroy platelets, therefore any newly transfused platelets will also be destroyed.

126. A) Henoch-Schonlein purpura (HSP) or anaphylactoid purpura is an immunoglobulin (IgA) mediated small blood vessel vasculitis that predominantly affects children but also is seen in adults. HSP is a subset of necrotizing vasculitis characterized by fibrinoid destruction of blood vessels and leukocytosis. Clinical presentations include, palpable purpura, arthralgia, or arthritis, abdominal pain, and gastrointestinal bleeding.

127. D) All are seen in haemolytic anaemia

a) Serum haptoglobin **reduced** not increased
b) Plasma methemalbumin present
c) Haemoglobinuria
d) Haemosiderinuria
e) Increased plasma haemoglobin
f) Increased serum bilirubin
h) Reticulocytosis
i) Spherocytosis

128. B) Pernicious anaemia is due to inadequate gastric production or defective function of intrinsic factor.

Hereditary lack of intrinsic factor may occur as autosomal recessive homozygous.

Autoimmune mechanism: Antibodies are present in the serum and gastric juice of most patients of pernicious anaemia.

Blocking antibodies block the binding of vitamin B_{12} to intrinsic factor and binding antibodies react with IF B_{12} complex and prevent it from binding to ileal receptors.

Histamine fast achlorhydria (Not hyperchlorhydria) and presence of IF antibodies in serum are detected.

The entire symptom complex of the tongue in pernicious anaemia is referred to as Hunter's glossitis or Moeller's glossitis. The tongue is sore, has a burning sensation, and shows atrophy of the papillae (beef streak).

Fissures and ulcers are common.

There is premature graying of hair.

Treatment is parenteral administration of vitamin B_{12}.

129. A) DIC does not occur in cases of diabetes.

Causes of DIC

I. **Infections**

- Gram negative bacteria: Meningococci, Enterobacteriacae, salmonella, Haemophilus, pseudomonas
- Gram positive bacteria: Pneumococci, staphylococci, haemolytic streptococci
- Anaerobes: Many species of clostridia, mycobacterium tuberculosis
- Fungi: Aspergillus, histoplasma, candida, Rickettsia-RMSF
- Protozoa: Malaria
- Other syndromes: Meningitis, Septic shock
- Post-splenectomy state, TSS

II. **Neoplasm**

- Haemopoietic: AML-M3, adult ALL (Philadelphia-positive ALL), CML etc.

- Solid: Many mucin secreting adenocarcinoma (pancreas, colon, ovary)

III. **Vascular disease:** Aortic aneurysm, giant haemangiomas, vascular tumours, Acute myocardial infarction, intracardiac tumour/thrombus vasculitis

IV. **Liver diseases**: Biliary obstruction, Reye's syndrome, fulminant hepatic failure, cirrhosis

V. **Obstetric complications:** Amniotic fluid embolism, placental abruption, various types of abortions, retained dead fetus, pregnancy induced hypertension, and molar pregnancy.

VI. **Transfusion reactions**

VII. **Venoms and strings:** Rattle snakes, vipers, cobra, scorpion, hymenoplera bites

VIII. **Injury and surgery:**

Crush injury

Burns: Hyperthermia, rhabdolysis, ischemia,/infarction,

Major surgery: Cardiac bypass, liver transplantation

Shock

RDS (respiratory distress syndrome) agents

IX. **Drugs and therapeutic agents:** Fibrinolytic, heparin, immune drug

X. Miscellaneous: Pancreatitis, acute intravascular haemolysis, sarcoidosis, anaphylaxis, Kawasaki disease, etc

130. B) B-cell chronic lymphocytic leukaemia B-CLL also known as chronic lymphoid leukaemia (CLL), is the most common type of leukaemia.

CLL affects B cell lymphocytes.

131. D) HAND SCHULLER CHRISTIAN DISEASE

A more localized variant, primarily referred to as Hand Schuller Christian disease, or multifocal eosinophilic granuloma is a childhood disease that consists of the triad of diabetes insipidus, lytic bone lesions. There are punched out lesions on X-ray and proptosis. It is the result of error of metabolism of cholesterol and its esters.

The age group involved is more than 3 years of age. It is more common in boys than girls 2:1.

Oral manifestations include:

1. Irregular ulceration of the hard palate, which may be the manifestation of the disease.
2. Gingival infiltration and ulcerated nodules, difficulty in chewing and foul smelling breath also occurs.
3. Loose and sore teeth with precocious exfoliation and failure of healing of tooth socket following extraction.

Microscopically: The lesion shows large number of foam cells, lymphocytes, plasma cells, eosinophils, neutrophils and an occasional giant cell. Langerhan's cells contain rod shaped cytoplasmic structure called as Birback granules.

132. C) Aleukaemic leukaemia: Aleukaemic leukaemia is characterized by a normal or low number of white blood cells in the blood despite leukaemic changes in tissues.

In aleukaemic leukaemia the total white blood cell count in **peripheral** blood is not elevated, it may be lymphocytic, monocytic, or myelogenous.

The term aleukaemic leukaemia is applied when there is proliferation of white blood cells in bone marrow but there are no abnormal cells in peripheral blood and the leukocyte count is normal or subnormal.

Indications of bone marrow biopsy

Anaemia

1. Hypoplastic and aplastic anaemia
2. Megaloblastic anaemia
3. Sideroblastic anaemia
4. Refractory anaemia

Leukaemia
1. Aleukaemic or subleukaemic leukaemia
Idiopathic thrombocytopaenic purpura
Multiple myeloma
Carcinoma
Collagen diseases.

133. B) Bone marrow biopsy is important to confirm the diagnosis of myelofibrosis.

Chronic idiopathic myelofibrosis, also known as Agogenic myeloid metaplasia (AMM) is a clonal myeloproliferative disease characterized by marrow fibrosis and splenomegaly due to extramedullary haemopoiesis.

Trephine biopsy: The bone trabeculae are markedly increased in size and number. Much of the haemopoeitic tissue is replaced by loose fibrous tissue. The haemopoietic tissue, though reduced in amount, is of normal appearance.

134. C) Chloroma a malignant, greenish neoplasm of myeloid tissue that occurs anywhere in the body of patients who have myelogenous leukaemia. The green pigment is primarily myeloperoxidase. The tumour tissue fluoresces bright red under ultraviolet light. It is also called granulocytic sarcoma.

135. D) Thromboembolism is not a complication of massive blood transfusion.

Storage of blood at 2-6° C for 48 hours is associated with loss of platelet function and labile coagulation factors. Coagulability is caused by a dilutional effect on host's clotting factors and platelets.

Circulatory overload: Following repeated transfusion, there is increased blood volume and venous pressure. In the elderly and pregnant women, cardiac function is affected. It is especially likely to occur and may result in acute pulmonary edema in patients with chronic severe edema and in patients with compromised cardiovascular function.

136. D) CPD-A anticoagulant is used for preservation of blood for blood transfusion.

137. D) Factor IX: Haemophilia B or Christmas disease is a clotting disorder caused by mutation of the factor IX gene. The factor IX gene is located on X-chromosome Xq 27.1—q 27.2. It is inherited as X-linked recessive. Mostly males are affected. It is second most common form of haemophilia. It is called Christmas disease after Stephen Christmas, the first patient described with this disease.

The factor IX deficiency leads to an increased prepotency for haemorrhage. This is in response to mild trauma or even spontaneously, such as in joints or muscles. Children with severe haemophilia B often begin to show increased prepotency for haemorrhage. This is in response to mild trauma or even spontaneously, such as in joints or muscles. Children with severe haemophilia B often begin to show increased bruising around the age of one year. It may present earlier if the child undergoes surgery, or after trauma, including immunization.

138. D) Massive blood transfusion is defined as replacement of the patient's total blood volume in less than 24 hours.

139. B) Glycosylated haemoglobin assay is helpful in the monitoring of patients with diabetes mellitus.

140. C) With acute blood loss if patient survives hypovolumic shock there occurs increased erythropoiesis. The marrow compensation or increased erythropoiesis is reflected by release of reticulocytes in the blood.

141. A) In megaloblastic anaemia the cells are macrocytic. Though cells synthesize their DNA but there is typically delay in mitotic division. Cytoplasm is all mature by this time but nuclei fail to divide and this immature situation is referred to as nuclear cytoplasmic asynchrony.

142. D) Fançoni's anaemia is a disease passed through families (inherited) that mainly affects the bone marrow. It results in decreased production of all types of blood cells.

Fanconi's anaemia is due to an abnormal gene that damages cells, which keeps them from repairing damaged DNA.

Persons with Fanconi's anaemia have lower than normal numbers of white blood cells, red blood cells, and platelets.

Thalassaemia major is known as **Cooley's anaemia.**

Gray baby syndrome is a rare but serious side effect that occurs in newborn infants following the intravenous administration of the antimicrobial chloramphenicol.

143. B) Thalassaemias are a diverse group of hereditary disorders in which there is reduced rate of synthesis of one or more of the globin polypeptide chain (alpha or beta chains)

144. D) Epstein-Barr virus infectious mononucleosis is also known as Pfeiffer's disease or kissing disease. Emil Pfeiffer described the syndrome as an infectious process in 1889.

The Paul-Bunnel test is positive in high dilutions, agglutinating the sheep's red blood cells due to the presence of heterophile antibody for EBV antigen.

145. A) von-Willebrand disease

Classic haemophilia is caused by a deficiency of only one of 3 components of factor VIII

von-Willebrand disease is caused by deficiency of all 3 components of factor VIII.

Factor VIII is a glycoprotein that has 3 components.

A. A clot promoting factor

B. Factor VIII antigen

C. von-Willebrand factor

Pseudohaemophilia, vascular haemophilia, vascular purpura

chapter 4

CARDIOVASCULAR PATHOLOGY

1. Anti-streptolysin O test is used in the diagnosis of:
   A) Rheumatoid arthritis
   B) Typhoid fever
   C) Rickettial fever
   D) Rheumatic fever
2. Harton's disease is
   A) Kawasaki disease
   B) Polyarteritis nodosa
   C) Temporal arteritis
   D) Wegner's granulomatosis
3. Saccular aneurysm occurs in:
   A) Atherosclerosis
   B) Syphilis
   C) All of the above
   D) None of the above
4. MacCallum patch is present in?
   A) Rheumatic endocarditis
   B) Myocardial infarction
   C) Giant cell myocarditis
   D) Viral myocarditis
5. MacCallum patch is present in?
   A) Rt. atrium
   B) Rt. ventricle
   C) Lt. atrium
   D) Lt. ventricle
6. PAN most commonly involve:
   A) Large vessel
   B) Medium and small arteries
   C) Arterioles
   D) Venules
7. Troponin T test is used in the diagnosis of:
   A) Cerebral infarction
   B) Myocardial infarction
   C) Pulmonary infarction
   D) Splenic infarction
8. Normal weight of heart is:
   A) 200 gram
   B) 300 gram
   C) 400 gram
   D) 500 gram
9. Normal thickness of Lt. ventricle is
   A) 8 mm
   B) 10 mm
   C) 15 mm
   D) 20 mm
10. Circumference of mitral valve is:
    A) 8 cm
    B) 9 cm
    C) 10 cm
    D) 12 cm
11. Normal capacity of Lt. atrium is:
    A) 20 ml
    B) 30 ml
    C) 40 ml
    D) 50 ml
12. Transmural infarct is common in:
    A) Rt. atrium
    B) Rt. ventricle

C) Lt. atrium
D) Lt. ventricle

13. Cardiomyopathy may be seen in all of the following except:
A) Duchenne muscular dystrophy
B) Friedreich's ataxia
C) Type I glycogen storage disease
D) Alkaptonuria

14. The tumour which most commonly metastasizes to heart is:
A) ALL
B) Non-Hodgkin's lymphoma
C) Bronchogenic carcinoma
D) Malignant melanoma

15. The tumour which commonly metastasizes to heart is:
A) Carcinoma stomach
B) Carcinoma breast
C) Carcinoma testis
D) Carcinoma ovary

16. Lipoprotein sub-fraction with the term "good" cholesterol is: associated
A) Very low-density lipoprotein (VLDL)
B) Low-density lipoprotein (LDL)
C) High-density lipoprotein (HDL)
D) Pre-beta lipoprotein

17. Most common cardiac tumour in children is:
A) Myxoma
B) Rhabdomyoma
C) Fibroma
D) Angioma

18. A patient with respiratory symptoms cough, haemoptysis and glomerulonephritis. His cANCA levels in serum is raised. Most likely diagnosis is:
A) Goodpasture syndrome
B) Classic polyarteritis nodosa
C) Wegner's granulomatosis
D) Kawasaki syndrome

19. "Thrush breast heart" or tigered heart is seen in:
A) Primary amyloidosis
B) Chronic venous congestion
C) Secondary amyloidosis
D) Fatty infiltration

20. Marantic endocarditis is associated with:
A) Malignancy
B) SLE
C) Carcinoid
D) Rheumatoid arthritis

21. Libman-Sacks endocarditis occurs in:
A) Rheumatic heart disease
B) SLE
C) Infective endocarditis
D) Carcinoid syndrome

22. Fatty streaks are first consistantly detected in arterial walls during which stage of life?
A) Children (8-14 years)
B) Young adults (21-30 yrs)
C) Middle age 31-40 yrs)
D) Older adults (41-60 yrs)

23. Lines of Zahn's are seen in:
A) Propogated clot
B) Primary platelet thrombus
C) Cordline thrombus
D) Post-mortem clot

24. Which of the following is not a clinical sign associated with bacterial endocarditis?
A) Kerning sign
B) Osler's node
C) Changing cardiac murmur
D) Roth's spots

25. Following are complications of mitral stenosis except:
A) Lt. atrium hypertrophy
B) Rt. ventricular hypertrophy
C) Lt. ventricular atrophy
D) CVC lung

26. All of the following may be seen in patients with cardiac temponade except:
A) Kussumal's signs
B) Pulsus paradoxicus
C) Electrical alterans
D) Rt. ventricular diastolic collapse on ECG

27. Specific marker for vascular endothelium is:
    A) Dohle bodies
    B) Weible palade bodies
    C) Asteroid body
    D) Schaumann bodies
28. Complications of myocardial infarction are except:
    A) Rupture of heart
    B) Cardiac aneurysm
    C) Myomalacia cordis
    D) Lt. ventricular atrophy
29. Aschoff body is the characteristic histological lesion of which of the following?
    A) Infective endocarditis
    B) Rheumatic endocarditis
    C) Marfan's syndrome
    D) Myocardial sarcoidosis
30. Causes of left ventricular hypertrophy are except:
    A) Hypertension
    B) Aortic stenosis
    C) Mitral stenosis
    D) Hypertrophic cardiomyopathy
31. Aortic incompetence is common in
    A) Gaucher's disease
    B) Tay-Sach's disease
    C) Ehler's-Danlos syndrome
    D) Marfan's syndrome
32. Contraction band necrosis in heart occurs in:
    A) Hypoxic injury due to shock
    B) Thrombosis
    C) Edema
    D) Amyloidosis
33. Softening of heart due to an infarct is known as:
    A) Cardiac tamponade
    B) Myomalacia cordis
    C) Post-myocardial infarction
    D) None of the above
34. Myomalacia cordis is a complication of:
    A) Myocardial infarct
    B) Rheumatic heart disease
    C) Toxic myocarditis
    D) Cardiomyopathy
35. Most common sites of spontaneous rupture of atherosclerotic aortic aneurysm is:
    A) Abdominal aorta above renal artery
    B) Arch of aorta
    C) Descending aorta
    D) Abdominal aorta below renal artery
36. Following are causes of dilated cardiomyopathy except:
    A) Alcohol associated cardiomyopathy
    B) Lt. ventricular decompensation
    C) Sarcoidosis
    D) Embryogenic non-compaction
37. Holiday heart syndrome is:
    A) Alcohol associated cardiomyopathy
    B) Amyloidosis of heart
    C) Hypertensive heart disease
    D) Glycogen storage disease
38. Following are causes of restrictive cardiomyopathy except:
    A) Glycogen storage disease type II
    B) Amyloidosis
    C) Myocarditis
    D) Endomyocardial fibrosis
39. Cause of dilated cardiomyopathy is
    A) Hypertension
    B) Tako-Tsubo-cardiomyopathy
    C) Tumours of heart
    D) Sarcoidosis
40. Which of these is responsible for atherosclerosis:
    A) Arginine
    B) Asparate
    C) Homocysteine
    D) Glycine
41. The predominant cell type of the inflammatory infiltrate in a 72 hours old myocardial infarction is:
    A) Lymphocyte
    B) Macrophages
    C) Polymorphonuclear leukocytes
    D) Fibroblast
42. Characteristic features of rheumatic heart disease is:
    A) Microabscess in myocardium

B) Fibrosis in endocardium
C) Valvular deformities
D) Papillary muscle fibrosis

43. Which is the most common type of pericarditis in rheumatic fever?
A) Serous
B) Purulent
C) Serofibrinous
D) Haemorrhagic

44. Most commonly affected artery in atherosclerosis:
A) Anterior descending branch of left coronary artery
B) Rt. coronary
C) Circumflex artery
D) Marginal artery

45. The most common cause of mitral stenosis in India is:
A) Rheumatic fever
B) Endocarditis
C) Congenital
D) Iatrogenic

46. Important change in benign hypertension in arterioles:
A) Fibrinoid necrosis
B) Microaneurysms
C) Thinning of walls
D) Hyaline arteriosclerosis

47. Pathological change in malignant hypertension is:
A) Hyperplastic arteriosclerosis
B) Cystic medial necrosis
C) Benign nephrosclerosis
D) Hyaline arteriosclerosis

48. Most common cause of aortic aneurysm is
A) Atherosclerosis
B) Trauma
D) Congenital
E) Acromegaly

49. Both systemic and pulmonary infarction is seen in:
A) Anterior wall MI
B) Posterior wall MI
C) Septal wall MI
D) Inferior wall MI

50. Following are found in association with Fallot's tetralogy except:
A) VSD
B) PS
C) Rt. sided aorta
D) PDA

51. Lt. ventricular hypertrophy is seen in all the conditions except:
A) Essential hypertension
B) Aortic stenosis
C) Aortic incompetence
D) Mitral stenosis

52. Most common cause of sustained severe hypertension in children:
A) Coarctation of aorta
B) Renal parenchymal disease
C) Aorta-arteritis
D) Pheochromocytoma

53. Tumours of blood vessels include all /EXCEPT
A) Glomus tumour
B) Angiosarcoma
C) Adenoma
D) Kaposi's sarcoma

54. Bacterial endocarditis is rarely seen in:
A) VSD
B) PDA
C) MVP
D) Ostium secundum ASD

55. Important features of Henoch Scholein purpura
A) Raised IgA
B) Membranous glomerulonephritis
C) Absent radial pulse
D) Aneurysm of branching point

56. Chronic constructive pericarditis is usually due to:
A) Lobar pneumonia
B) Myocardial infarction
C) Tuberculosis
D) SLE

57. Bacterial endocarditis can cause all except:
   A) Cerebral infarcts
   B) Focal glomerulonephritis
   C) Meningitis
   D) Subcutaneous nodes
58. Which is not a feature of benign hypertension in kidney?
   A) Hyaline arteriosclerosis
   B) Interstitial lobular fibrosis
   C) Medial hypertrophy of small vessels
   D) Fibrinoid necrosis
59. Osler's nodes are pathognomic of:
   A) Subacute bacterial endocarditis
   B) Rheumatoid arthritis
   C) Rheumatic fever
   D) Thrombocytopaenia
60. Myocardial infarction most often result in:
   A) Mitral stenosis
   B) Aortic regurgitation
   C) Aortic stenosis
   D) Mitral regurgitation
61. Raynaud's phenomenon is seen in all except:
   A) Atherosclerosis
   B) Scleroderma
   C) Buerger's disease
   D) Juvenile arthritis

Answers

1. D) Antistreptolysin O titre: Titre of anti-streptolysin O antibodies is a blood test used to assist in the diagnosis of a streptococcal infection. The ASOT test helps to direct the antimicrobial treatment and is used in the diagnosis of scarlet fever, rheumatic fever and post-infectious glomerulonephritis.

2. C) Harton's disease is a headache syndrome characterized by inflammation of the temporal (temporal arteritis) and other cranial arteries. A pulseless, enlarged superficial artery and a severe throbbing headache are the principal symptoms. Systemic manifestations include anorexia, insomnia, weight loss, and low-grade fever. Occurs in old age group (7th and 8th decade) seldom before age 55; affects both sexes equally.

3. C) Saccular aneurysm represents a sac like dilatation, which bulges from one side of the artery and may be connected to it by a small aperture. It is seen in atherosclerosis and syphilis.

4. A) MacCallum patch is seen in chronic rheumatic heart disease.

5. C) It is a focus of rough wrinkled endocardium in the posterior aspect of the left atrium, which serves as a clue to previous rheumatic involvement.

6. B) Polyarteritis nodosa is a vasculitis of medium and small sized arteries, which becomes swollen and damaged from attack by rogue immune cells.

7. B) Certain subtypes of troponin (cardiac troponin I and T) are very sensitive and specific indicator of damage to the heart muscle myocardium. They are measured in the blood to differentiate between unstable angina and myocardial infarction. Troponin test is reliable above serum level of > 0.10 ng/ml. In myocardial infarction (up to 8 hours) troponin-T is important since it usually becomes positive after 4 hours. At this time sensitivity and specificity of troponin test is 100% and 80% respectively.

8. B) Normal weight of the heart in males is 280 to 340 grams and in females 230 to 280 grams.

9. C) Normal thickness of wall of left ventricle is 13 to 15 mm.

10. C) Normal circumference of mitral valve is 10 cm.

11. C) Normal capacity of left atrium is 40 ml. It is more than 400 ml in mitral stenosis.

12. D) Transmural infarct—involving the entire thickness of the left ventricular wall from endocardium to epicardium, usually the anterior free wall and posterior free wall and septum with extension into the RV wall in 15-30%. Isolated infarcts of RV and Rt atrium are extremely rare.

13. B) Dilated cardiomyopathy occurs in type I glycogen storage disease, alkaptonuria, and Duchenne muscular dystrophy.

14. C) Metastatic tumours: Lung and breast carcinoma, soft tissue sarcoma and renal cancer are the most common sources of metastasis to the heart. Malignant melanoma, leukaemia, and lymphoma often metastasize to the heart, but the metastases may not be clinically significant.

15. B) Same as 14.

16. C) It is hypothesized that HDL can remove cholesterol from atheroma within arteries and transport it back to the liver for excretion or reutilization, which is the main bound cholesterol is sometimes called "good cholesterol"

17. B) Rhabdomyomas are hamartomas and are the most frequently found tumours in children. They are associated with tuberous sclerosis in 50 to 80% of cases. These tumours are frequently multiple involving ventricular free and septal walls and have yellowish grey colour. They vary from small to extremely large.

18. C) Antineutrophilic cytoplasmic antibodies: Typically ANCA are demonstrated by immunoflouresence testing of patient's serum incubated with ethanol-fixed normal human neutrophils. Almost all patients with active systemic Wegner's granulomatosis have a positive ANCA commonly directed against PR3. Approximately 80-90% of all ANCA found in patients with Wegner's granulomatosis are c-ANCA/anti PR3.

19. D) Fatty change is more often patchy than diffuse; the myocardium shows parallel brown bands of unaffected muscle fibres alternating with yellow bands of muscles loaded with fat. This striated appearance is known as "Thrush breast appearance or Tiger stripping appearance".

20. A) Non-bacterial thrombotic endocarditis (NBTE) or marantic endocarditis is most commonly found on previously undamaged valves. The vegetations are small, sterile, and tend to aggregate along the edges of the valve or the cusps. NBTE usually occurs in patients with cancers, particularly mucinous adenocarcinoma of lung, stomach, and pancreas.

21. B) Libman-Sacks endocarditis is a form of non-bacterial endocarditis that is seen in systemic lupus erythematosus. It is one of the most common cardiac manifestations of lupus.

22. A) Early proliferative or fatty streak phase: Fatty streaks and dots are the earliest deposits of lipid in the intima of the aorta and larger arteries are seen predominantly in childhood (8 to 14 years).

23. B) Cardiac and. arterial thrombus are formed slowly in rapid circulation. They are pale-grey and tend to have gross and microscopic lamination (lines of Zahn) produced by pale layers of platelets and fibrin alternating with darker red cell rich layers. These are mostly seen in the left ventricle overlying an infarct.

24. A) Oslers nodes are painful small swelling 1 cm or so appear at the tip of the fingers or toes in 20% of cases and so called Osler's nodes after eminent Canadian physician Sir William Osler. They are believed to be a manifestation of hypersensitivity vasculitis. Embolism of central artery of the retina may cause canoe shaped haemorrhagic spots with pale center called Roth's spot.

25. A) Complications of mitral stenosis include left atrial dilatation, right ventricular hypertrophy, left ventricular atrophy, pulmonary hypertension, chronic venous congestion of lung, embolism, CVC kidney, infarction, brain, limbs, kidney, and spleen.

26. D) Cardiac tamponade is a condition involving compression of the heart caused by blood or fluid accumulation in the space between the myocardium and pericardium. The blood or fluid collects within the pericardium. This prevents the ventricles from expanding fully so they cannot adequately fill or pump blood. Kussmaul sign is usually observed in patients with constrictive pericarditis and cardiac tamponade. Electrical alternans associated with pericardial effusion is strongly suggestive of impending or established cardiac tamponade. Other signs of tamponade include pulsus paradoxius (a drop of at least 10 mm Hg in arterial blood pressure on inspiration.

27. B) Weible palade bodies are storage granules of endothelial cells, the cells that form the inner lining of the blood vessels and heart. They store and release two principal molecules, von-Willebrand factor and P-selectin, and thus play a dual role in haemostasis and inflammation.

Dohle body is a discrete round, or oval body found in neutrophils and associated with infections, burns, trauma, pregnancy or cancer.

An Asteroid body is a histological finding seen in granulomatous disease such as sarcoidosis and foreign body giant cell reactions. Schaumann bodies are basophilic, lamellated, shell-like (conchoidal) bodies found in the cytoplasm of multinucleated giant cell of granulomas.

28. D Complications of myocardial infarction include ventricular arrhythmias, cardiogenic shock, mural thrombosis with embolism, rupture of heart, myomalacia cordis, mitral incompetence, and cardiac aneurysm.

29. B) The Aschoff nodule or bodies are pathognomic of rheumatic carditis. Aschoff bodies, named after German pathologist (1866-1942), begin to appear a few weeks after the onset of rheumatic carditis and persist in the heart for months or years. Aschoff bodies are fusiform or spheroidal, usually 200 to 600 μm across. The Aschoff body is found typically in the myocardium but may also be seen in the endocardium, and pericardium.

30. C) Causes of left ventricular hypertrophy include, aortic stenosis, hypertension, hypertrophic cardiomyopathy. Mitral stenosis causes atrophy of left ventricle.

31. D) A sign of regurgitation from prolapse of aortic valve results from cystic medial degeneration of the valves, which is commonly associated with Marfan's syndrome. Marfan's syndrome is caused by defects in gene called fibrillin-1. Fibrillin-1 plays an important role as the building block for elastic tissue in the body.

32. A) The earliest change histologically seen with hypoxic injury due to shock is contraction band necrosis. The myocardial fibres are beginning to loose cross striations and the nuclei are not visible in most of the cells.

33. B) Softening of heart due to an infarct is known as myomalacia cordis.

34. A) Large infarct shows softening of muscle (myomalacia cordis) leading to rupture and death.

35. D) Most common site of rupture of atherosclerotic aortic aneurysm is abdominal aorta below the level of renal artery.

36. C) Causes of dilated cardiomyopathy are as follows?

1. Idiopathic
2. Alcohol abuse
3. Major catecholamine discharge (Tako-Tsubo cardiomyopathy)
4. Myocarditis
5. Post-partum cardiomyopathy
6. Doxourabicin
7. Endocrinopathies
8. Genetic diseases
9. Left ventricular decompensation
10. Inherited disorders –Muscular dystrophy

11. Embryogenic non-compaction
12. Glycogen storage diseases type IV (Anderson's disease)

37. A) Alcohol–associated cardiomyopathy: Acute or chronic consumption of excessive quantities of alcohol are associated with myocardial damage. Concentric ventricular hypertrophy and systemic hypertension are common accompaniments of this syndrome also known as the Holiday heart syndrome. Microscopic examination of heart will show edema of vasculature and mitochondria.

38. C) Causes of restrictive cardiomyopathy are as follows:

1. Amyloidosis
2. Post-radiation
3. Post-operative surgery
4. Diabetes
5. Endomyocardial fibrosis and Loffler's syndrome
6. Sarcoidosis
7. Tumours of heart
8. Glycogen storage disease type II (Pomp's disease)

39. B) Tako-tsubo cardiomyopathy, also known as transient apical ballooning, apical ballooning cardiomyopathy, stress induced cardiomyopathy, broken heart syndrome. Tako-tsubo is the Japanese name for octopus traps that fishermen still use to catch octopus. The shape that the left ventricle takes (Tako-tsubo) is due to a state of complete exhaustion of the heart muscle.

Several cases of interesting cardiomyopathy have been reported in Japan, United States, and Belgium.

Pathogenesis

The pathogenesis of this disorder is not well understood but several mechanisms have been proposed.

1. Transient vasospasm: Some of the original researchers of Tako-tsubo suggested that multiple simultaneous spasms of coronary arteries could cause enough loss of blood flow to cause transient stunning of the myocardium.
2. Microvascular dysfunction: The theory going the traction is that there is dysfunction of the coronary arteries at the level where they are no longer visible by coronary angiography.
3. It has been described following some stressful events, such as hypoglycemia, lightning strikes, earthquakes, post-ventricular tachycardia, during alcohol withdrawal, following surgery, during hyperthyroidism and following emotional stress.

Complications

Acute complications of stress-induced cardiomyopathy can include tachyarrhythmias, bradyarrhythmia, pulmonary edema, mitral regurgitation, and cardiogenic shock.

40. C) Evidence suggests that homocysteine may promote atherosclerosis by damaging the inner lining of arteries and promoting blood clots.

41. C) In 24-72 hours total loss of nuclei, and striations along with heavy neutrophilic infiltrate occurs in myocardium in myocardial infarction.

42. C) Characteristic feature of rheumatic heart disease is rheumatic valvulitis.

Mitral valve is most commonly and severely affected (65-70%), and aortic valve is second in frequency (25%). The tricuspid valve is deformed in only 10% of patients and almost always is associated with mitral and aortic lesion. The pulmonary valve is rarely affected.

Microabscesses can occur when septic emboli lodge in the coronary circulation often as a consequence of infective endocarditis.

In some cases of myocardial infarction papillary muscle undergoes necrosis, followed by organization and fibrosis, sometimes accompanied by stretching and various degrees of persistent regurgitation.

43. C) Serofibrinous pericarditis is the common type of pericarditis in rheumatic fever.

Gross: Exudate is small in amount consisting mainly of fibrin which is deposited on both the surfaces of the pericardium giving it a typical shaggy of bread and butter appearances. The fibrin may glue the pericardial surfaces together and is removed by the process of organization which results in fibrous thickening and often permanent adhesion of the layers with partial or complete obliteration of the sac. About 10% of patients with rheumatic fever develop a pericardial friction rub or a pericardial effusion.

Microscopically: Fibrin covers the surface of pericardium and infiltration of lymphocytes, histiocytes and plasma cells is prominent. Occasionally, fibrinoid necrosis with Aschoff bodies may be seen in acute rheumatic fever. On recovery exudate is completely absorbed but a portion of it may become organized and fibrosed forming opaque white patch called **milk spot.** There is calcification with formation of stony plates on the surface of the heart.

44. A) Arteries involved

1. Anterior descending branch of left coronary artery (40 to 50% cases) areas affected are anterior wall of left ventricle, apex and anterior 2/3rd of interventricular septum
2. Right coronary artery (30 to 40% cases): It involves inferoposterior wall of the left ventricle, posterior 1/3rd of interventricular septum.
3. Circumflex branch of left coronary artery. (15 to 20% cases) Area involved is lateral wall of left ventricle and part of posterior wall of right ventricle.

45. A) The most common cause of mitral stenosis in India is rheumatic fever.

Other causes are:

- Congenital
- Malignant carcinoid
- Systemic lupus erythematosus
- Rheumatoid arthritis
- Mucopolysaccharidosis

46. D) **Hyaline arteriosclerosis:** Small arteries and arterioles show hyaline degeneration. It is characterized by acidophilic thickening of the subintimal tissue; but later it involves the entire thickness of arterial wall with obliteration of lumen. Changes are best seen in kidney and retina. Hyaline arteriosclerosis leads to endothelial damage, exudation of plasma proteins into the smooth muscle layers of the arterioles, increase ECM deposition in the arterioles. The muscular media is converted to an eosinophilic hyaline structure.

47. A) Arteriosclerosis, often described as a thickening and hardening of the arteries, appears in various forms and can be related to a number of different causes. Hyperplastic arteriosclerosis is characterized by a pattern of thickening commonly linked to an onion- skin, concentric laminations of smooth muscle cells and basement membranes being deposited on top of the other in layers. As more and more layers are added, the luminal space of the affected artery is progressively narrowed. Hyperplastic arteriosclerosis is often linked with malignant hypertension and frequently affects blood vessels of the kidneys, though it can occur anywhere.

48. A) The most common cause of aortic aneurysm is atherosclerosis. The aneurysms are more common in males after the age of 50 years. They are fusiform or saccular. They are 15 cm in greatest diameter and of variable length. Most commonly occur in abdominal aorta, arch of aorta, common iliac artery, renal artery and mesenteric artery.

Pathogenesis: The aneurysm forms as a result of weakening and thinning of media underlying atheromatous ulcer.

Microscopically: Wall of aneurysm consists of all the layers of aorta. There is atheroma with marked leukocytic infiltration, and fatty debris, later on perianeurysmal lymphocytic infiltration, macrophages, giant cells and fibrosis.

Effects

1. **Rupture:** The aneurysm may rupture while still small, into peritoneal cavity with retroperitoneal or intraperitoneal haemorrhage causes acute surgical abdominal emergency. It gives rise to potentially fatal haemorrhage.
2. **Arterial occlusion:** Aneurysmal sac is nearly filled with the thrombus causing ischaemia of leg either by occluding the iliac arteries. Obstruction of mesenteric, renal or vertebral arteries (supplying the spinal cord) occurs by mural thrombus or embolus from atheroma.
3. Abdominal aortic aneurysm causes compression of ureter or erosion. Impingement of vertebrae, on an adjustment structures such as into peritoneal cavity. It presents as pulsatile abdominal mass that simulates a tumour.

49. C) Infarction occurs due to emboli from a thrombus formation due to ventricular wall immobility. In septal Myocardial infarction there is immobility wall of both right ventricle and left ventricle as septum is common to both. Right ventricle thrombus leads to emboli in pulmonary vasculature and left thrombus leads to emboli in systemic vasculature.

50. D) **A. PS:** A narrowing of the right ventricular outflow tract can occur at the pulmonary valve (pulmonary stenosis PS) or just below the pulmonary valve (infundibular stenosis). Stenosis is mostly caused by overgrowth of the heart muscle wall (hypertrophy of the septoparietal trabeculae). An aortic valve with biventricular connection, that is, it is situated above the ventricular septal defect and connected to both the right and left ventricle.

B. Overriding of aorta: The aortic root can be displayed the front (anteriorly) or directly above the septal defect, but it is always abnormally located to the right of the root of the pulmonary artery.

C. VSD: A hole between the two bottom chambers (ventricles) of the heart. The defect is centered around the most superior aspect of the ventricular septum and in the majority of the cases is single and large.

D. Rt. ventricular hypertrophy: Right ventricle is more muscular than normal, causing a characteristic boot shaped (Coeur-en-sabot) appearance as seen by chest X-ray.

Additional anomalies

1. Stenosis of the left pulmonary artery in 40% of patients.
2. A bicuspid pulmonary valve in 40% of patients.
3. Right sided aortic arch in 25% of patients.
4. Coronary artery anomalies, in 10% of patients.
5. A foramen ovale or atrial septal defect, which cause the syndrome is sometimes called a pentalogy of Fallot.
6. An atrioventricular septal defect
7. Partially or totally anomalous pulmonary venous return
8. Forked ribs and scoliosis

51. D) In cases of mitral stenosis left ventricle is atrophic.

Causes of left ventricular hypertrophy include:

1. Aortic stenosis
2. Essential hypertension
3. Aortic incompetence

52. B) Most common cause of sustained severe hypertension in children is renal parenchymatous disease.

Causes of hypertension in children

1. Glomerulonephritis
2. Obstructive uropathy
3. Reflux nephropathy
4. Thrombotic microangiopathy
5. Renovascular disease
6. Coarctation of aorta
7. Hypoplastic/dysplastic kidney
8. Takayasu's arteritis (aorta-arteritis)
9. Renal artery stenosis
10. Pheochromocytoma

53. C) Adenoma is a benign tumour arising from glandular epithelium.

Vascular tumours include:

Haemangioms
Glomus tumour
Haemangioendothelioma, haemangiopericytoma
Angiosarcoma
Kaposi's sarcoma

54. D) Ostium secundum defect represents the persistence of foetal foramen ovale. Because of the greater distensibility of the right atrium, blood flows from left to right through the defect. This allows recirculation of blood through the lungs and back to the left side of the heart.

If undetected the complications include:

1. Heart failure: Chronic volume loading of the right side of the heart leads to cardiac failure at some time during adult life. This complication may be precipitated by atrial fibrillation or flutter.
2. Pulmonary hypertension

55. A) Henoch-Scholein purpura is a systemic hypersensitivity disease of unknown cause characterized by a purpuric rash, colicky abdominal pain, polyarthralgia and acute glomerulonephritis. There is acute glomerulonephritis not membranous glomerulonephritis. There is deposits of IgA and fibrin in the mesangial regions of glomeruli. Serum levels of IgA are raised in Henoch-Schloein purpura.

56. C) Constructive pericarditis is due to progressive thickening, fibrosis, and calcification of the pericardium. The condition often follows an attack of tuberculous pericarditis but can also complicate haemopericardium., viral pericarditis, rheumatoid arthritis, purulent pericarditis, radiation therapy, cardiac surgery and histoplasmosis. The affected pericardium may be so thick (up to 3 cm) that obliterates the pericardial space and is seen as a rigid mass of fibrous tissue, which narrows the orifice of venae cavae. Fibrous pericarditis constricts the cardiac chambers, particularly reducing right atrial filling. Elevation of jugular venous pressure and decreased cardiac output results. Surgical removal of thickened pericardial sac (pericardicectomy) is effective treatment.

Symptoms are dyspnoea, chronic edema, hepatic congestion and ascitis. Atrial fibrillation is common.

Pericardial plaques

Serous pericarditis: This condition is caused by noninfectious inflammation such as rheumatoid arthritis (RA) and systemic lupus erythematosus (SLE).

Fibrinous pericarditis: The type of pericardial reaction may result from bacterial, viral or other infections, rheumatic fever, myocardial infarction, irradiation to the chest, uremia and tuberculosis.

57. C) Symptoms are due to lesions, which are divided in to three groups.

1. Cardiac lesions

Valvular lesions: Characterized by sterile vegetations comprised of platelet, and fibrin thrombi on one or more cardiac valves. Most commonly the mitral and aortic valves are involved. Rarely other valves may be affected. The lesion is proliferative than destructive. These vegetations are generally large varying from 1 to

5 mm and are projecting on the surface of the valve cusps.

2. Embolic lesions

I. **Skin:** Osler nodes are painful small swellings 1cm or so appear at the tip of the fingers or toes in 20% of the patients and are called Osler's node after the eminent Canadian physician Sir William Osler. They are believed to be a manifestation of hypersensitivity vasculitis.

II. Petechiae may appear usually in small numbers and splinter haemorrhages under the nails. Petechiae may be caused by emboli, but more likely due to toxic damage to the capillaries or hypersensitivity vasculitis caused by the lodgment of immune complexes in small vessels in the dermis.

III. **Kidneys**: Petechial haemorrhages are seen on the surface of the kidney, giving a flea bitten appearance. Focal glomerulonephritis develops in about 30% of cases. Diffuse glomerulonephritis is much less common. Infarction may occur in many cases due to blocking of terminal arteries.

IV. Spleen may become palpable. There is formation of infarction in the spleen characterized by pain in that organ.

V. **Brain**: In the brain, the emboli usually cause only transient neurological dysfunction. It may lead to infarction and hemiplegia.

VI. **Retina**: Embolism of central artery of the retina may cause canoe shaped haemorrhagic spots with a pale center called Roth's spot.

VII. **Intestine**: Infarction of intestine.

3. **General**: Cardiac failure and toxemia: There is cellular swelling and fatty changes in the liver and kidney. It causes subacute combined degeneration of spinal cord and splenomegaly with anaemia.

58. D) Fibrinoid necrosis; Fibrinoid necrosis affects mainly the distal portions of the interlobular arteries and the afferent arteriole.

Hyaline arteriosclerosis: Small arteries and arterioles show hyaline degeneration. It is characterized by acidophilic thickening of the subintimal tissue; but later it involves the entire thickness of arterial wall with obliteration of lumen. Changes are best seen in kidney and retina. Hyaline arteriosclerosis leads to endothelial damage, exudation of plasma proteins into the smooth muscle layers of the arterioles, increase ECM deposition in the arterioles. The muscular media is converted to an eosinophilic hyaline structure.

Larger interlobular arteries: The intimal thickening may narrow the interlobular arteries.

59. A) Osler nodes are painful small swellings 1cm or so appear at the tip of the fingers or toes in 20% of the patients and are called Osler's node after the eminent Canadian physician Sir William Osler. They are believed to be a manifestation of hypersensitivity vasculitis.

60. D) Most often complication of myocardial infarction is mitral incompetence. It is due to rupture of papillary muscles.

61. D) Common causes of Raynaud's phenomenon are:

1. Diseases of arteries: Such as atherosclerosis, Buerger's disease, which is associated with smoking.
2. Drugs that cause narrowing of arteries such as amphetamines, certain types of betablockers, some cancer drugs, Ergot compounds, and methyl sergide.
3. Arthritis and autoimmune conditions: Scleroderma, Sjogren's syndrome, rheumatoid arthritis, and systemic lupus erythematosus.
4. Repeated injury.
5. Smoking.
6. Frostbite.
7. Thoracic outlet syndrome.

chapter 5

PULMONARY PATHOLOGY

1. Pseudobronchiectasis is seen in:
   A) Lung abscess
   B) Atelectasis
   C) Bronchopneumonia
   D) Emphysema
2. Ghon focus can be appreciated in:
   A) Primary tuberculosis
   B) Secondary tuberculosis
   C) Miliary tuberculosis
   D) Progressive tuberculosis
3. Which of the following symptoms are rare in patients with progressive lung cancer?
   A) Haemoptysis
   B) Hypercalcaemia
   C) Headache
   D) Urinary retention
4. Invasive aspergillosis can be diagnosed by examination of:
   A) Sputum
   B) Blood culture
   C) Brushing
   D) An open lung biopsy
5. Which of the following is the most common primary lung tumour in infants and children?
   A) Pulmonary blastoma
   B) Squamous cell carcinoma
   C) Endobronchial carcinoma
   D) Metastatic osteogenic carcinoma
6. Ferruginous bodies result in:
   A) Sarcoidosis
   B) Silicosis
   C) Tuberculosis
   D) Asbestosis
7. Pleural calcification is seen in:
   A) Asbestosis
   B) Silicosis
   C) Anthracosis
   D) Byssinosis
8. Amyloidosis can commonly complicate the following except
   A) Bronchiectasis
   B) Chronic bronchitis
   C) Fibrocaseous tuberculosis
   D) Lung abscess
9. Egg shell calcification is seen in all except:
   A) Silicosis
   B) Bronchogenic carcinoma
   C) Lymphoma
   D) Sarcoidosis
10. Characteristic lesion of pulmonary aspergillosis is:
    A) Interstitial fibrosis
    B) Emphysema
    C) Granulomas
    D) Psammaoma bodies
11. In a coal minor aged 50 years a persistent blood stained pleural effusion is most likely to be due to
    A) Pulmonary tuberculosis
    B) Coal miner's pneumoconiosis

C) Carcinoma of lung
D) Silicosis

12. Pulmonary thromboembolism arises from:
A) Deep leg vein
B) Renal vein
C) Cerebral vein
D) Veins of upper limb

13. Bronchiectasis is most common in which lobe?
A) Rt. upper lobe
B) Middle lobe
C) Lt. lower lobe
D) Lt. upper lobe

14. Pulmonary infiltrated with eosinophilia encompass all of the following except:
A) Allergic bronchopulmonary aspergillosis
B) Chronic eosinophilic pneumonia
C) Loffler's syndrome
D) Extrinsic allergic alveolitis

15. Accumulation of carbon pigment in tissue of lung produces:
A) Anthracosis
B) Silicosis
C) Asbestosis
D) Byssinosis

16. Pulmonary embolus is seen in:
A) Main pulmonary artery
B) Bifurcation of pulmonary artery
C) Rt. pulmonary artery
D) Lt. pulmonary artery

17. Granulomas seen in lung in all conditions except:
A) Sarcoidosis
B) Berylliosis
C) Tuberculosis
D) Asbestosis

18. Caplan syndrome consists of the following:
A) Silicosis + tuberculosis
B) Pneumoconiosis + Rheumatoid arthritis
C) Byssinosis
D) Asbestosis +tuberculosis

19. Cavity containing masses in lung are:
A) Aspergillosis
B) Tuberculosis
C) Hydatid cyst
D) All of the above

20. Which of the following disease is caused by Thermoactinomycosis vulgaris?
A) Farmer's lung
B) Byssinosis
C) Bagassosis
D) Anthracosis

21. Hamann-Rich disease is:
A) Usual interstitial pneumonia
B) Desquamative interstitial pneumonia
C) Respiratory bronchiolitis
D) Acute interstitial pneumonia

22. Which type of carcinoma of lung causes Horner's syndrome?
A) Squamous
B) Oat cell
C) Adenocarcinoma
D) Large cell

23. Primary pleural tumour is
A) Mesothelioma
B) Myxoma
C) Lipoma
D) Fibroma

24. Exposure to cotton dust in a textile factory causes:
A) Bagassosis
B) Byssinosis
C) Anthracosis
D) Silicosis

25. The causes of cor pulmonale include all the following except:
A) Lung abscess
B) Emphysema
C) Bronchiectasis
D) Silicosis

26. Common anterior mediastinal tumours are except:
A) Thymoma
B) Teratoma
C) Neurogenic tumours
D) Lymphoma

27. Commnest tumour of posterior mediastinum is:
A) Thymoma
B) Lymphoma
C) Neurogenic
D) Teratoma

28. The most common termination of lobar pneumonia is:
A) Consolidation
B) Resolution
C) Abscess formation
D) Empyema

29. Brown induration of lung is seen in:
A) Silicosis
B) Siderosis
C) Asbestosis
D) Bagassosis

30. Which statement is correct in Goodpasture's syndrome?
A) Necrotizing haemorrhagic interstitial pneumonitis
B) Alveolitis
C) Patchy consolidation
D) Pulmonary edema

31. Alpha 1 antitrypsin deficiency occurs in:
A) Emphysema
B) Bronchogenic carcinoma
C) Empyema
D) Bronchiectasis

32. Brewer's lung is seen in:
A) Aspergillosis
B) Sarcoidosis
C) Tuberculosis
D) Histoplasmosis

33. Curschmann's spirals in sputum is seen in:
A) Tuberculous cavity
B) Bronchial asthma
C) Bronchitis
D) Bronchiectasis

34. Charcot-Leyden crystals are seen in all except:
A) Bronchial asthma
B) Parasitic lesions of lung
C) Allergy
D) Bronchiectasis

35. Most common cause of respiratory distress after birth in first 24 hours is:
A) Neonatal sepsis
B) Meconium aspiration
C) Pneumonia
D) Air embolism

Answers

1. B) Pseudobronchiectasis is a condition in which bronchiectasis like pattern is present and appears in the bronchogram of partially atelectatic pulmonary segments. When the large bronchi have become shortened and broadened in outline, these reversible changes do not indicate destruction of the bronchial wall.

2. A) A Ghon focus is a primary lesion caused by mycobacterium bacilli (tubercle bacilli) developed in the lung of a previously uninfected individual. The lesions consist of a calcified focus of infection and an associated lymph node. Gross appearance there is a small tan-yellow subpleural granuloma in the mid-lung field on the right. In the hilum is a small yellow tan granuloma in a hilar lymph node next to a bronchus.

3. D) Symptoms in progressive lung cancer are haemoptysis, pain due to pleurisy, pressure nerves and metastasis in the vertebral column, headache, dysphagia, hypercalcaemia, dysponea, and cyanosis.

4. D) When systemic aspergillosis is associated with skin lesions, the diagnosis is simple by histological examination.

5. A) Primary lung neoplasms are rare in children. Most common primary lung malignancies in children are pleuropulmonary blastoma, and carcinoid tumour. Other primary paediatric lung tumours include congenital peribronchial myofibroblastic lesions, sarcomas, carcinomas and mesothelioma.

6. D) Ferruginous body is a histologic finding in interstitial lung disease suggestive of significant asbestos exposure (asbestosis). They appear as small brown nodules in the septum of the alveolus. Ferruginous bodies are fibres of asbestos coated with an iron rich material derived from proteins such as ferritin and haemosiderin.

7. A) Exposure to asbestos can lead to focal plaque like pleural fibrosis at times with calcification, occurring up to 20 year after the initial exposure.

8. B) Cases with bronchiectasis, fibrocaseous tuberculosis, and lung abscess cause generalized secondary amyloidosis of adrenal, liver, and kidney.

9. B) Egg shell calcification is seen in sarcoidosis, silicosis, coal- worker's pneumoconiosis, berylliosis, Hodgkin's lymphoma, histoplasmosis, amyloidosis, blastomycosis, and scleroderma.

10. A) Interstital fibrosis is the result of exposure to high concentrations of airborne asbestos fibres for approximately 10-20 years and although found in more than 50% of heavily exposed workers. Bronchiolar fibrosis may be the first and early manifestations of asbestosis. Pulmonary reaction consists of a widespread interstitial type of fibrosis, which is accompanied by diaphragmatic pleural calcification.

11. C) Haemorrhagic pleural effusion is common in carcinoma lung. Adenocarcinoma of lung is commonly associated with pleural effusion. In this case coal worker must be suffering from carcinoma lung. In coal worker's pneumoconiosis and silicosis there is no pleural effusion. In cases of tuberculosis pleural fluid is clear not haemorrhagic.

12. A) Pulmonary embolism is a blockage of the main artery of the lung or one of its branches by a substance that has travelled from elsewhere in the body through the blood stream. Usually this is due to embolism of a thrombus from the deep veins in the legs a process termed venous thromboembolism.

13. C) The posterior basal segment of left lower lobe is affected most often.

14. D) In extrinsic allergic alveolitis there is no infiltration of lung by eosinophils. Blood examination shows eosinophilia. Pulmonary diseases associated with eosinophilia are heterogeneous group disorders. They include Loffler's syndrome, Dress syndrome, schistosomiasis, allergic bronchopulmonary aspergillosis, and acute and chronic eosinophilic pneumonia.

15. A) Accumulation of carbon particles in lung tissue is known as anthracosis. Byssinosis, also called "Brown lung disease" or "Monday fever" is an occupational lung disease caused by exposure to cotton dust in inadequately ventilated work environment. Silicosis and asbestosis is caused by inhalation of silica and asbestos respectively.

16. A) Pulmonary embolus is seen in main pulmonary artery before bifurcation into right and left pulmonary artery.

17. D) Granulomatous lesions of lungs include sarcoidosis, tuberculosis, atypical mycobacterial infection, histoplasmosis, coccidioidomycosis, cryptococcus, blastomycosis, actinomycosis, pneumocystitis carinii silicosis, chronic berylliosis and coal worker's pneumoconiosis. Berylliosis is caused by inhalation of metal beryllium.

18. B) Caplan syndrome is a combination of rheumatoid arthritis, and pneumoconiosis, that manifests as intrapulmonary nodules which appear as homogenous and well-defined on chest X-ray. Caplan syndrome occurs in patients with both rheumatoid arthritis, and pneumoconiosis, related to mining dust (coal, asbestos, silica). The condition occurs in miners (especially those working in anthracite coal mines), asbestosis, silicosis and other pneumoconiosis.

19. D) Cavity containing masses in lung is:

C. Carcinoma: Squamous cell carcinoma

A. Autoimmune: Wegner's granulomatosis, rheumatoid nodules

V. Vascular: Emboli (septic and bland)

I. Infection. Bacterial pneumonia, fungal pneumonia, pneumatocele, lung abscess and hydatid cyst

T. Trauma. Pulmonary laceration

Y. Young. Congenital. Congenital cystic adenomatoid malformation, pulmonary sequestration, bronchogenic cyst

20. A) Farmer's lung is extrinsic allergic alveolitis or hypersensitivity alveolitis. Bagassosis is a hypersensitivity pneumonitis due to inhalation of dust from bagasse (the residue of cane after extraction of sugar). Byssinosis, also called "Brown lung disease" or "Monday fever" is an occupational lung disease caused by exposure to cotton dust in inadequately ventilated work environment. Anthracosis is caused by deposition of coal particles in lungs.

21. D) Acute interstitial pneumonitis is clinically known as Hamann-rich syndrome. Wide age range, many young patients. Acute onset of dyspnoea followed by rapid development of respiratory failure. Half of patients report a viral syndrome preceding lung disease.

Pathologic changes reflect acute response to injury within a days or weeks. Fibrosis and minimal collagen deposition.

22. A) The most common cell type causing Horner's syndrome is squamous cell carcinoma. Direct invasion by the tumour of anatomic structures can cause functional syndromes. For instance, phrenic nerve infiltration can cause diaphragmatic paralysis; an upper lobe tumour can invade into the lower cervical sympathetic plexus and upper thoracic nerve roots that form the lower part of the brachial plexus. This induces a peculiar telltale syndrome of severe pain in the distribution of the ulnar nerve, and ipsilateral enophthalamos, ptosis, miosis, and anhidrosis.

23. A) Mesothelioma is a primary neoplasm arising from mesothelial cells lining the pleural cavity.

This malignancy is associated very strongly with asbestos exposures. Approximately 50% of the patients have a history of exposure to asbestos.

Macroscopically: Pleural mesothelioma characteristically encases and compresses the lung, extending into fissures and interlobar septa. Areas of necrosis within the tumour give rise to large cystic spaces containing mucinous fluid.

Microscopically:

1. Epithelial, in which cuboidal cells line tubular and microcystic spaces, into which small papillary buds project.
2. Predominantly fibrous mesothelioma is made up of fine spindle cells arranged in whorls and straps.
3. Combination of two.

These are highly malignant tumours that spread around the pleural cavity and pericardium, encasing the lung and mediastinal structures.

Spread: Pleural mesotheliomas tend to spread locally within the chest cavity, invading and compressing major structures. Metastasis can occur to the lung parenchyma, and mediastinal lymph nodes, as well as to extrathoracic sites such as the liver, bones, periosteum, and adrenals.

Clinical features: The average age of patients with mesothelioma is 60 years. Patients are first seen with pleural mass, chest pain, and nonspecific symptoms, such as weight loss and malaise.

24. B) Bagassosis is a hypersensitivity pneumonitis due to inhalation of dust from bagasse (the residue of cane after extraction of sugar). Byssinosis, also called "Brown lung disease" or "Monday fever" is an occupational lung disease caused by exposure to cotton dust in inadequately ventilated work environment. Anthracosis is caused by deposition of coal particles in lungs.

Silicosis is due to inhalation of silica particles.

25. A) Cor pulmonale or pulmonary heart disease is enlargement of the right ventricle of the heart as a response to increased resistance or high blood pressure in the lungs (pulmonary hypertension)

Causes of cor-pulmonale include:
1. Chronic obstructive pulmonary disease
2. Chronic blood clots in the lungs
3. Cystic fibrosis

26. C) Neurogenic tumours are common in posterior mediastinum.

Anterior mediastinal tumours are:
1. Thymoma
2. Thymic carcinoid
3. Germ cell tumours
4. Lymphoma
5. Haemangioma
6. Parathyroid carcinoma
7. Thymic cyst
8. Aberrant thyroid
9. Lymphangioma

27. C) Commonest tumour of posterior mediastinum is neurogenic tumours.

Tumours of posterior mediastinum include:
1. Neurofibroma
2. Neurilemmoma
3. Neurofibrosarcoma
4. Ganglioma
5. Ganglioneuroblastoma
6. Neuroblastoma
7. Paraganglioma pheochromocytoma

28. B) Resolution begins on eighth day.

Macroscopically: Lung is friable, edematous, mottled or red in colour with many foci of liquefication. Proteolytic enzymes liquefy fibrin to produce granular, semi fluid debris that is reabsorbed, ingested by macrophages, or coughed out. Since there is virtually no tissue destruction in lobar pneumonia, the lung parenchyma returns to normal,

Complications

1. Organisation: In organized or unresolved pneumonia there is failure of the mechanism of liquefaction and absorption of the exudate. Instead the exudate is organized by granulation tissue. The fibrous tissue formed is seen to be continuous from one alveolus to another through the pores of Kohn.
2. Pleural effusion: About 5% of treated cases of lobar pneumonia develop inflammation of pleura with effusion.
3. Empyema: Suppurative material may accumulate in the pleural cavity producing an empyema.
4. Lung abscess is a complication, which has practically disappeared since the introduction of antibiotic. In untreated cases organisms that result in larger tissue necrosis lead to suppuration. This is typically seen in Staphylococcal pneumonia, as well as in many Gram negative and of course in fungal pneumonia.
5. Cardiac complications include myocarditis, pericarditis, endocarditis, peripheral circulatory failure, and venous thrombosis.
6. Bacteraemia: Nonspecific complications are due to toxaemia and anoxia. They are: paralytic ileus due to loss of tone of bowel muscle; jaundice due to haemolysis of red cells in the local lesion and possibly due to hepatic dysfunction.
7. **Joint arthritis.**

29. B) Brown induration is fibrosis and haemosiderin pigmentation of lungs due to long standing chronic venous congestion of lungs.

The condition is characterized by firmness of the lungs, and a brown colour associated with haemosiderin-pigmented macrophages in alveoli, consequent upon long continued congestion due to heart disease.

30. A) Goodpasture's syndrome is characterized by rapidly progressive glomerulonephritis and haemorrhagic interstitial pneumonitis. In cases of Goodpasture's syndrome the lungs are heavy, focal necrosis of alveolar wall, fibrous thickening of septa with mild hyperplasia of alveolar lining cells, organization of blood in alveolar space and haemosiderin laden macrophages and linear deposits of immunoglobulin along basement membrane.

31. A) Alpha 1 antitrypsin deficiency: Alpha 1 antitrypsin is a proteolytic enzyme inhibitor, which protects the lung against an elastase (HNE) released from neutrophils. This is synthesized in liver and the production is increased during inflammatory or infective conditions. Tobacco smoke inhibits the release of AIMT from the macrophages. The elastase in absence of AIMT carries out its destructive action. Children with deficiency of AIAT suffer from emphysema and cirrhosis of liver.

32. A) Pulmonary aspergillosis

Aspergillus is a ubiquitous fungus, which may cause an allergic pulmonary response to otherwise healthy individuals. This is known colloquially as Bewer's lung and belongs to a group of diseases known by the term extrinsic allergic alveolitis.

33. B) **Curschumann's spirals:** They are yellowish white spirally twisted masses of mucus occurring in sputum in bronchial asthma. They may be seen in fresh sputum under low power and may be visible by naked eye.

34. D) **Charcot Leyden crystals:** They vary in size and may be as large as 50 µm in length. Charcot Leyden crystals are slender and pointed at both ends, consisting of a pair of hexagonal pyramids joined at their bases.

They are indicative of a disease involving eosinophilic inflammation or proliferation, such as is found in allergic reactions and parasitic infections. Charcot Leyden crystals are often seen pathologically in patients with bronchial asthma.

35. B) Meconium aspiration syndrome usually occurs in post mature and small for dates babies.

Clinical findings-usually develop respiratory distress in first 24 hours of life if untreated leads to respiratory failure.

Complications

1. Pneumothorax
2. Air leak syndrome
3. Pneumopericardium
4. Pneumomediastinum
5. Persistent pulmonary hypertension

X-ray shows hyperinflation, patchy infiltrates

chapter 6

RENAL PATHOLOGY

1. Nephrotic syndrome is characterized by all except:
   A) Massive albuminuria
   B) Increased blood urea
   C) Normal blood pressure
   D) Increased serum cholesterol
2. Disease associated with multiple, recurrent renal calculi is:
   A) Cystinuria
   B) Homocystinuria
   C) Alkaptonuria
   D) None
3. Focal glomerunephritis is associated with all except:
   A) Fanconi's syndrome
   B) SLE
   C) Bacterial endocarditis
   D) Henoch-Schonlein purpura
4. Wilm's tumour is characterized by chromosomal aberrations:
   A) 11 P
   B) 11q
   C) 13P
   D) 13q
5. Most common presentation of Wilm's tumour is:
   A) Haematuria
   B) Hydronephrosis
   C) Abdominal mass
   D) Abdominal pain
6. Commonest type of glomerulonephritis causing nephritic syndrome in children is:
   A) Crecentric glomerulonephritis
   B) Membranoproliferative glomerulonephritis
   C) Minimal change disease
   D) Focal segmental glomerulonephritis
7. The immune mechanism mediating Goodpasture's syndrome is:
   A) Type I hypersensitivity reaction
   B) Type II reaction
   C) Type III reaction
   D) Anaphylactic reaction
8. Von-Hansemann cells are characteristics of:
   A) Cytomegalovirus infection
   B) Malakoplakia
   C) Xanthogranuloma pyelonephritis
   D) None of the above
9. IgA nephropathy is seen in:
   A) Membranous glomerulonephritis
   B) Mesangioproliferative G
   C) Focal glomerulonephritis
   D) Crescentic glomerulonephritis
10. Contracted granular kidney is seen in.
    A) Chronic pyelonephritis
    B) Chronic glomerulonephritis
    C) Benign nephrosclerosis
    D) All of the above
11. Large white kidney is seen in:
    A) KW lesion

B) Benign nephrosclerosis
C) Malignant nephrosclerosis
D) Chronic pyelonephritis.

12. The antigen in Goodpasture's syndrome is:
A) Unknown
B) A globular non-collagenous domain of collagen IV:
C) An organic inhalant
D) Denatured DNA

13. Large white kidney is seen in:
A) KW lesion
B) Lipoid nephrosis
C) Amyloidosis
D) All of the above.

14. Flea bitten kidney is seen in:
A) Malignant nephrosclerosis
B) Subacute glomerulonephritis
C) Post-streptococcal glomerulonephritis
D) All of the above

15. Renal pathology in SLE is all except:
A) Lipoid nephrosis
B) Focal proliferative
C) Diffuse proliferative
D) Diffuse membranous

16. Wilm's tumour has been linked to which of the following tumour syndromes?
A) WAGR syndrome
B) Denys-Drash syndrome
C) Beckwith syndrome
D) All of the above.

17. Haematuria is least likely to occur in :
A) Transitional cell carcinoma pelvis
B) Renal tubular adenocarcinoma
C) Acute post streptococcal GN
D) Urinary lithiasis

18. Armani Ebstein lesion is seen in:
A) Diabetes mellitus
B) Lipoid nephrosis
C) Chronic pyelonephritis
D) Acute streptococcal glomerulonephritis

19. Papillary necrosis is most frequent in:
A) Diabetes mellitus
B) Acute pyelonephritis
C) Sickle cell anaemia
D) Analgesic nephropathy

20. Renal artery stenosis may occur in all of the following except:
A) Atherosclerosis
B) Fibromuscular dysplasia
C) Takayasu's arteritis.
D) Polyarteritis nodosa

21. Hydronephrosis is associated with all of the following except:
A) Benign prostatic hyperplasia
B) Acute cystitis
C) Normal pregnancy
D) Tumours

22. Common cause of Nephrotic syndrome in adults is:
A) Lupus nephritis
B) Diabetes
C) Amyloid
D) Drugs

23. Crescentic glomerulonephritis is:
A) Acute GN
B) RP GN
C) Membranous GN
D) MPGN

24. CPN is most commonly caused by:
A) Post-streptococcal
B) Reflux nephropathy
C) Analgesic nephropathy
D) Diabetic nephropathy

25. Feature of membranous glomerulonephritis.
A) Diffuse capillary wall thickening
B) Hypercellular glomeruli
C) Subendothelial deposits
D) Neutrophil infiltration of glomerular tuft

26. Acute tubular necrosis occurs in
A) Renal edema
B) Amyloidosis
C) Shock
D) KW lesion

27. Following parasites causes nephrotic syndrome except:
   A) Plasmodium malariae
   B) Schistosoma mansoni
   C) Leishmania donovani
   D) Ascaris lumbricoides
28. Painless haematuria occurs in:
   A) Nephrolithiasis
   B) Tuberculosis of kidney
   C) Renal cell carcinoma
   D) Cystitis
29. Following are features of chronic pyelonephritis except:
   A) Hypertension
   B) Specific gravity 1.025
   C) Polyuria
   D) Anaemia
30. Following are renal changes in diabetes except:
   A) KW lesion
   B) Papillitis necroticans
   C) Armani Ebstein lesion
   D) Flea bitten kidney
31. Low complement levels are seen in following conditions except:
   A) Idiopathic proliferative glomerulonephritis
   B) Crescentic glomerulonephritis
   C) IgA nephropathy
   D) Membrano-proliferative glomerulonephritis
32. Normal complement level is seen in following conditions except:
   A) Goodpasture's syndrome
   B) Lupus nephritis
   C) Henoch-Scholein purpura
   D) Microscopic polyarteritis nodosa
33. Following are causes of azotemia except:
   A) GIT bleeding
   B) Liver disease
   C) Acute glomerulonephritis
   D) Acute interstitial nephritis
34. Which of the following does not complicate acute pyelonephritis
   A) Pyonephrosis
   B) Papillitis necroticans
   C) Renal cell carcinoma
   D) Perinephric abscess
35. Following are characteristics of Fanconi syndrome except:
   A) Aminoaciduria
   B) Hyperkalemia
   C) Glucosuria
   D) Excess bicarbonate loss and metabolic acidosis
36. Heymann nephritis antigen is seen in:
   A) Rapidly progressive glomerulonephritis
   B) Focal segmental glomerulonephritis
   C) Membranous glomerulonephritis
   D) IgA nephropathy
37. Bad prognostic factor for crescentic glomerulonephritis is:
   A) Number of glomeruli
   B) Size of glomeruli
   C) Cellularity
   D) Rupture of basement membrane
38. The common renal lesions in diabetes mellitus:
   A) Papillary necrosis
   B) Fibrin cap in the glomerulus
   C) Nodular sclerosis of the basement membrane
   D) Diffuse thickening of basement membrane
39. Staghorn calculus is associated with:
   A) Oxalate calculi
   B) Urate calculi
   C) Phosphate calculi
   D) Cystine calculi
40. Main cause of edema in nephrotic syndrome is:
   A) Loss of potassium
   B) Loss of solutes
   C) Hypoproteinaemia
   D) Derrangements of fatty acids

41. The endocrine manifestation, which may occur in renal cell carcinoma
   A) Cushing's syndrome
   B) Gynaecomastia
   C) Renin related hypertension
   D) Peptic ulcer
42. Cause of renal failure in septicaemic shock is:
   A) Acute tubular necrosis
   B) Acute cortical necrosis
   C) Glomerulonephritis
   D) Focal necrosis
43. Causes of painless haematuria in Children include all of the following except:
   A) Acute glomerulonephritis
   B) Renal calculus
   C) IgA nephropathy
   D) Wilm's tumour
44. Occupations at risk for bladder cancer include all of the following except:
   A) X-ray technicians
   B) Textile workers
   C) Petrol workers
   D) Paints
45. The following glomerular lesions are associated with hepatitis B infection except:
   A) Membranous glomerulopathy
   B) IgA nephropathy
   C) Polyarteritis nodosa
   D) Crescentic glomerulonephritis
46. Spider leg appearance of calyces on intravenous urography is seen in:
   A) Congenital cystic kidneys
   B) Hypernephroma
   C) Horseshoe kidney
   D) Hydronephrosis
47. Wilm's tumour is associated with all/ except
   A) Hemihypertrophy
   B) Anirida
   C) Backwith-Wiedmann's syndrome
   D) Polycystic kidney
48. WBC cast in urine are seen in:
   A) Amyloidosis
   B) Chronic glomerulonephritis
   C) Acute pyelonephritis
   D) Hypernephroma
49. Wilm's tumour commonly metastasize to:
   A) Lung
   B) Lymph nodes
   C) Brain
   D) Liver
50. Transitional cell carcinoma can be caused by:
   A) Napthylamine
   B) Smoking
   C) Bilharziasis
   D) Betel nut
51. In which of the following conditions bilateral contracted kidneys are characteristically seen:
   A) Amyloidosis
   B) Diabetes mellitus
   C) Rapidly progressive glomerulonephritis
   D) Benign nephrosclerosis
52. Bilateral contracted kidneys occur in all except:
   A) Diabetes
   B) Benign nephrosclerosis
   C) Chronic pyelonephritis
   D) Chronic glomerulonephritis
53. Bloody brown casts are found in:
   A) Acute glomerulonephritis
   B) Acute tubular necrosis
   C) Idiopathic crescentic glomerulonephritis
   D) Lipoid nephritis
54. The manifestations of chronic renal failure include all of the following Except:
   A) Hypertension
   B) Uraemic pericarditis
   C) Secondary hyperthyroidism
   D) Massive proteinuria

Answers

1. **B)** Nephrotic syndrome is characterized by massive albuminuria, massive oedema, increased serum cholesterol, normal blood pressure and normal blood urea.

2. **A)** Cystinuria is an autosomal recessive defect in resorptive transport of cystine and the diabetic amino acids ornithine, arginine, and lysine from the luminal fluid of the renal proximal tubule and small intestine. The only phenotypic manifestation of cystinuria is cystine urolithiasis, which often recurs throughout an affected individual's life.

3. **A)** Focal glomerulonephritis may be an early or mild manifestation of SLE, polyarteritis nodosa. Henoch-Schonlein purpura, Goodpasture's syndrome, subacute bacterial endocarditis, and Wegner's granulomatosis.

4. **A)** Wilm's tumour or nephroblastoma is cancer of the kidneys that typically occurs in children, rarely in adults. Mutation of the WT gene on chromosome 11p13 are observed in approximately 20% of Wilm's tumour. The tumour is caused by loss of inactivation of a tumour suppressor gene called WT1 on chromosome 11.

5. **C)** Most common presentation of Wilm's tumour is abdominal mass.

6. **C)** Minimal change disease is the commonest glomerulopathy in children. It is also known as lipoid nephrosis.

7. **B)** The immune mechanism mediating Goodpasture's syndrome is type II hypersensitivity reaction. Formation of IgG and IgM, which binds to the antigen or target cell surfaces, leading to phagocytosis of target cells by C8 C9 fraction of the activated complement.

8. **B)** Von-Hansemann cells are large histiocytic cells with abundant clear, granular cytoplasm associated with numerous intra and extracellular laminated and calcified spherules, the Michelis-Gutmann bodies. These are seen in malakoplakia.

9. **B)** **IgA** nephropathy is mesangioproliferative glomerulonephritis. Membranous glomerulonephritis causes nephritic syndrome. Crescentic glomerulonephritis causes nephritic syndrome and it is rapidly progressive glomerulonephritis.

10. **D)** Contracted granular kidneys are small in size. Surface is granular. There is decortication. Cut surface shows thinning of cortex. Contracted granular kidneys are seen in chronic pyelonephritis. Chronic glomerulonephritis, benign nephrosclerosis, and late stages of amyloidosis.

11. **A)** Nodular glomerulosclerosis or intercapillary glomerulosclerosis—This is peculiar to diabetic patients and found in 15% cases. The deposits may be discrete-rounded nodules, sometimes laminated, situated near the tip of the lobule and therefore appearing peripheral in the glomerulus ('Kimmelsteil Wilson lesion'). Many nodules are present within single glomeruli and most glomeruli become involved. The deposits are positive on periodic acid Schiff staining. Nodular glomerulosclerosis can give rise to Nephrotic syndrome.

12. **B)** It is believed to be type II hypersensitivity reaction to Goodpasture's antigen on the basement membrane of the glomerulus of the kidneys and pulmonary alveolus, specifically the non-collagenous domain of alpha-3 chain of Type IV collagen.

13. **D)** Large white kidneys are increased in size and weight, white in colour. Outer surface is smooth. On cutting there is no demarcation between cortex and medulla. Causes of large white kidneys include: Membranous glomerulonephritis, diabetic glomerulosclerosis, amyloidosis, systemic

lupus erythematosus, lipoid nephrosis, and focal segmental glomerulosclerosis.

14. D) Gross appearance of flea bitten kidney: On removal of capsule red spots are seen on the surface of the kidney. Causes of flea bitten kidney include acute post streptococcal glomerulonephritis, malignant nephrosclerosis, subacute bacterial endocarditis, Polyarteritis nodosa, and Wegner's granulomatosus. Henoch-Scholein purpura, and Goodpasture's syndrome.

15. A) In systemic lupus erythematosus kidneys show minimal mesangial lupus nephritis, mesangial proliferative lupus nephritis, focal proliferative lupus nephritis, diffuse proliferative nephritis, membranous lupus nephritis and advanced sclerosing lupus. Lipoid nephrosis gives rise to nephritic syndrome.

16. D) The syndromes associated with WT 1 abnormalities Wilm's tumour are:

1. WAGR syndrome acronym of Wilm's tumour, aniridia, genital abnormalities, mental retardation, shows a much higher risk of Wilm's tumour than general population.
2. Dany's Drash syndrome: Inter sexual disorders and glomerulopathy.
3. Backwith-Wiedemann syndrome

17. D) In cases of acute post streptococcal glomerulonephritis there is microscopic haematuria. Carcinoma of renal pelvis, renal tubular adenocarcinoma and urinary lithiasis are associated with massive haematuria.

18. A) Armani-Ebstein lesion: Glycogen accumulation occurs in tubular epithelial cells and is seen in the diabetic who has had marked hyperglycemia and glycosuria. It is also known as glycogen infiltration or glycogen nephrosis. It is glycogen infiltration with vacuolization of the tubular epithelium in convoluted tubules especially in distal tubules and loop of Henle.

19. D) Renal papillary necrosis is a disorder of kidney in which all parts of renal papilla die. The etiology of renal papillary necrosis includes diabetes, analgesic abuse or overuse, sickle cell disease, pyelonephritis, renal vein thrombosis, tuberculosis, and obstructive uropathy. Renal papillary necrosis is most commonly associated with analgesic nephropathy.

20. D) Renal artery stenosis is the narrowing of renal artery, most often caused by atherosclerosis, fibrous dysplasia, arteritis, renal artery aneurysm, extrinsic compression, (e.g., neoplasm), neurofibromatosis and fibrous band.

21. B) Hydronephrosis is caused by benign prostatic hypertrophy, normal pregnancy, tumours, and posterior urethral valves. Other causes include stones in the ureter, and compression of ureter by bands of fibrous tissue.

22. B) In adults most common cause of nephrotic syndrome is diabetic glomerulosclerosis. Other causes include membranous glomerulonephritis, amyloidosis, drug induced, and SLE.

23. B) Rapidly proliferative glomerulonephritis is also known as crescentic glomerulonephritis. The majority of glomeruli show formation of crescent. It is initiated by passage of fibrin into the Bowman's space as a result of increased permeability of glomerular basement membrane.

24. B) Most common cause of chronic pyelonephritis is reflux nephropathy. Chronic pyelonephritis occurs in patients with major anatomic abnormalities, such as obstructive uropathy, kidney stones.

25. A) Membranous nephropathy is a kidney disorder caused by diffuse thickening of capillary basement membrane.

26. C) Acute tubular necrosis is a kidney disorder involving damage to the tubule cells of the kidneys, resulting in acute kidney failure. Acute tubular necrosis is caused by hypotension and hypovolaemic shock following trauma, burns, or haemorrhage. There is rapid fall in blood pressure, which causes hypoperfusion of the peritubular capillaries and consequent tubular necrosis along the entire length of the nephron. The kidney appears pale and swollen.

Histology reveals infiltration of inflammatory cells and the tubular cells. The tubular cells are flattened and vacuolated. There is interstitial edema and cellular debris and protein casts in the distal tubules and the collecting ducts.

27. D) Nephrotic syndrome is recognized with parasitic infestations include Schistosoma mansoni, plasmodium malariae, leishmania donovani, trypanosomiasis, taenia echinococcus, toxoplasma gondii, and woucheria bancrofti.

28. B) Painless haematuria occurs in cases of tuberculosis. Causes of painful haematuria include: Nephrolithiasis, renal cell carcinoma, cystitis, schistosomiasis, carcinoma of renal pelvis and bladder.

29. B) Specific gravity of urine is low and fixed (1010). Anaemia is present in all the patients. Anaemia is due to chronic infection. There is polyuria. Patient complains of mild discomfort and dull pain in renal area. There are irregularities in the form of increased frequency, urgency and dysuria. Hypertension is present in half of the cases.

30. D) Renal lesions in diabetes include Armani Ebstein lesion, KW glomerulosclerosis, chronic pyelonephritis, atherosclerosis of renal artery, and papillitis necroticans.

31. C) In IgA nephropathy complement level is normal. In cases of idiopathic proilferative glomerulonephritis, membranoproliferative glomerulonephritis and crescentic glomerulonephritis complement level is low.

32. B) In lupus nephritis complement level is low. Normal complement level is seen in Goodpasture's syndrome, Henoch-Scholein purpura, and microscopic polyarteritis nodosa.

33. B) Blood urea is decreased in cases of liver diseases. Other causes of low blood urea are malnutrition and excessive alcohol consumption.

Causes of azotemia (high blood urea)

A. Prerenal causes

1. Absolute decrease in relative volume
   - Haemorrhage due to trauma
   - Gastrointestinal bleeding
   - Loss of plasma in burns
   - Crush injuries
   - Renal fluid loss (diuretics, diabetes)
2. Relative decrease in blood volume
   - Congestive cardiac volume
   - Dehydration
   - Septic shock
3. Arterial occlusion
   - Thrombosis of arteries
   - Occlusive embolism of aorta or renal arteries

B. Intrarenal azotemia

1. Renovascular obstruction

   Renal artery obstruction, atherosclerotic plaque, malignant hypertension, eclampsia
2. Glomerulus: Acute glomerulonephritis

3. Tubules: Tubular necrosis due to ischaemia, drugs or toxins
4. Acute interstitial nephritis due to infection or drug reaction
5. Nephrosis from precipitation crystals or protein

C. Post-renal azotemia

1. Ureteric: Calculi, blood clot, cancer
2. Bladder neck: Neurogenic bladder, prostatic hyperplasia, calculi, cancer, blood clot.
3. Urethra: Stricture, congenital valve, phimosis.

34. C) Complications of acute pyelonephritis are:

1. Gram-negative sepsis with shock,
2. Pyonephrosis,
3. Perinephric abscess,
4. Papillitis necroticans
5. Emphysematous pyelonephritis

35. B) Fanconi's syndrome is a disease of the proximal renal tubules of the kidney in which glucose, amino acids, uric acid, phosphate and bicarbonate are passed into the urine, instead of being reabsorbed. The clinical features of renal tubular acidosis are polyuria, polydipsia, hypophosphatemic rickets and osteomalacia, growth failure, acidosis, hypokalemia and hyperchloremia.

36. C) A complex of antigenic proteins obtained from the brush border of kidney tubules. It contains two principal components LDL-receptor related protein 2 and LDL receptor associated protein. The name of this complex is derived from researcher, Dr Walter Heymann who developed an experimental model of membranous glomerulonephritis by injecting this antigenic complex into rats to induce an autoimmune response.

37. A) Crescents are formed by proliferation. The prognosis can be roughly related to the number of crescents: Patients with crescents in less than 80% of glomeruli have a slightly better prognosis than those with higher percentages of crescents.

38. C) Five important lesions are encountered.

1. Armani Ebstein lesions
2. Glomerulosclerosis
3. Renal vascular lesion
4. Chronic pyelonephritis
5. Papillitis necroticans

Armani Ebstein lesion— It is glycogen infiltration with vacuolization of the tubular epithelium in convoluted tubules especially in distal tubules and loop of Henle.

Glomerulosclerosis—This consists of deposition of eosinophilic hyaline material in the mesangium of the glomerular lobule. Glomerulosclerosis may be nodular or diffuse.

Nodular glomerulosclerosis or intercapillary glomerulosclerosis: This is peculiar to diabetic patients and found in 15% cases. The deposits may be discrete rounded nodules, some times laminated, situated near the tip of the lobule and therefore appearing peripheral in the glomerulus ('Kimmelsteil Wilson lesion'). Many nodules are present within single glomeruli and most glomeruli become involved. The deposits are positive on periodic acid Schiff staining. Nodular glomerulosclerosis can give rise to Nephrotic syndrome.

Diffuse glomerulosclerosis: The glomerular capillary basements are thickened throughout their entire length. Obliteration of most of the capillaries and severe hyalinization of the glomeruli occurs.

Fibrin cap: Fibrin cap is an exudative lesion characterized by homogenous bright red crescentic deposit in a capillary of a peripheral lobule. The deposit is trapped on either side of basement membrane between endothelial cells and capillary basement membrane or between capillary basement membrane and visceral epithelial cells of the Bowman's capsules. **Capsular drops** are focal thickening of the parietal epithelial layer of Bowman's capsule. This is eosinophilic and drop hangs into the Bowman's capsular space. The capsular drop is PAS positive.

Renal vascular lesions and arteriosclerosis: Atheroma is very common and often severe in diabetes produce ischaemia, progressive scarring and contraction of kidney.

Chronic pyelonephritis: Pyelonephritis is an acute or chronic inflammation of the kidneys occurs in diabetics due to high blood sugar level and more chance of infection.

Necrotising papillitis: The acute type of glomerulonephritis with necrotising papillitis is proved to develop in diabetes. It may give rise to acute fatal renal failure and haematuria.

39. C) Sometimes a very large calculus nearly fills the calyces system, with extension into calyces that give the appearance of a stag's (dear) horns. Hence the name is "staghorn calculus".

Staghorn calculi are composed of struvite (magnesium ammonium phosphates) and are usually seen in the setting of infection with urease producing bacteria (e.g., proteus, klebsiella, pseudomonas, and enterobacter).

Struvite amounts for approximately 70% of these calculi, and is usually mixed with calcium phosphates.

40. C) In nephrotic syndrome, the glomeruli become damaged due to inflammation and hyalinization so that small proteins such as albumin, immunoglobulins and antithrombin can pass through the kidneys in to urine. According to the classical underfill hypothesis, there is persistent and heavy loss of plasma proteins, particularly albumin, in the urine. Hypoalbuminemia causes reduced oncotic pressure of plasma proteins and decreased ingoing of fluid from interstitium, which leads to edema.

As the concentration of proteins in the plasma falls, reducing the osmolality of the plasma, water moves from the blood into the tissues, causing hypovolemia and edema.

41. A) Renal cell carcinoma has been found to account for 2% of all neoplasm that are responsible for Cushing's syndrome. Although rare, Cushing's syndrome in RCC is believed to occur secondary to enzymatic conversion of pro-opiomelanocortin (POMC) to ACTH by tumour. The ectopic ACTH then drives cortisol secretion by adrenal glands. The diffuse adrenal hyperplasia seen in these cases appears to support this hypothesis.

42. A) Acute tubular necrosis (ATN) is caused by lack of oxygen to the kidney tissues (ischaemia of the kidneys). The internal structures of the kidney tissue particularly the tissues of the kidney tubule become damaged and destroyed.

ATN is one of the most common causes of kidney failure in hospitalized patients. Risk of acute tubular necrosis include:

1. Blood transfusion reaction
2. Injury or trauma that damages muscles.
3. Recent major surgery
4. Septic shock or other forms of shock

5. Severe low blood pressure (hypotension) that lasts longer than 30 minutes.
6. Liver and kidney damage in diabetes (diabetic nephropathy) make a person susceptible to the condition.

ATN can be caused by:

- Exposure to medications that are toxic to kidneys (such as aminoglycoside antibiotics)
- Antifungal agents (Amphotericin)
- Dye used for X-ray

43. B) **Causes of painful haematuria in children include**:

1. Urinary tract infection
2. Renal calculus

Causes of painless haematuria in children

Glomerular diseases
IgA nephropathy
Acute glomerulonephritis
Hydronephrosis with or without trauma
Polycystic disease of kidney
Tuberculosis of kidney
Schistosomiasis
Wilm's tumour

44. A) X-ray radiation causes leukaemia.

Chemicals: Bladder cancer has proven to have occupational basis-affecting workers under sustained exposure to aniline dyes, textiles, leather, paint, organic chemicals (petrol) and rubber. The provocative agents are 4-aminobiphenýl betanaphthylamine, benzine, and 4-nitrobiphenyl compounds.

45. D) Infection with hepatitis B virus (HBV) may be associated with a variety of renal diseases. HBV-related nephropathy is one of the HBV infection with extrahepatic manifestations.

Several morphological patterns for glomerular lesions have been described including:

1. Membranous nephropathy,
2. Membranoproliferative glomerulonephritis
3. Mesangial proliferative glomerulonephritis
4. Polyarteritis nodosa
5. Minimal change disease
6. IgA nephropathy
7. Focal glomerulonephritis

Many patients are asymptomatic, with plasma serology positive for hepatitis B surface antigen (HbsAg), hepatitis core antibody, and hepatitis B antigen (HbsAg). The pathologic role of HBV in these processes has been documented primarily by demonstration of hepatitis B antigen-antibody complexes in renal lesions.

Renal disease associated with hepatitis B virus infection

Lesion	Clinical presentation	Pathogenesis
Membranous nephropathy	Nephritic syndrome	Deposition of HbeAg with anti-HBeAb
Polyarteritis nodosa	Vasculitis Nephritic	Deposition of circulating antigen antibody complexes
Membranoprolifetative glomerulonephritis	Nephritic syndrome Nephrotic syndrome	Deposition of complexes containing HbeAg, HBsAg

46. A) The characteristic IVP and renal angiographic findings may confirm the diagnosis of polycystic kidney. IVP findings like spider leg appearance and sponge-like nephrographic effect can produce crescentic deformities of calyces (wind glass sign) may also be seen

47. D) Polycystic kidney is not associated with Wilm's tumour

A. Both kidneys are equally affected, the incidence of bilateral involvement being 5 to 10 percent.

B. Nephroblastoma arises within the substance of the kidney. Tumour is well-circumscribed, rounded, bosselated and soft in consistency

C. In its classic form it is without a definite capsule

D. Size is extremely variable, with a median 500 grams. It may vary from 500 to 2500 grams.

E. Invasion by tumour thrombus of the veins is frequently obvious to the naked eye

Cut section shows solid and pale gray or tan, fleshy white and often exhibits areas of cystic changes, necrosis and haemorrhage. Lobular pattern resulting from fibrous septation is common. Multicentric foci are appreciable in 70%. The syndromes associated with WT-1 abnormalities are:

1. **WAGR syndrome** acronym of Wilm's tumour, aniridia, genital abnormalities, and mental retardation, shows a much higher risk of Wilm's tumour than the general population. Children with WAGR syndrome revealed a deletion in the short arm of one copy of chromosome 11 (11p13)

   A second gene for susceptibility to Wilm's tumour (WT2) was discovered in sporadic tumours.
2. Denys-Drash syndrome (DDS) Intersexual disorders, glomerulopathy.
3. Backwith-Wiedemann syndrome

48. C. Pus cells (white blood cell) casts

1. Indicative of inflammation or infection
2. Pyelonephritis
3. Acute allergic interstitial nephritis
4. Nephritic syndrome
5. Post-streptococcal glomerulonephritis

They indicate suppurative lesions in kidneys.

They form by aggregation of pus cells/leukocytes in renal tubules.

49. A) Lung is the most common site of metastasis in Wilm's tumour. The tumour can be very large and it may metastasize to other body tissue.

Once the tumour has penetrated the renal capsule it spreads rapidly to involve the omentum and juxtarenal tissues. Invasion of the adrenal gland is common and frequently the neoplasm directly infiltrates the liver, intestines or vertebrae. The regional lymph nodes are often involved and metastasis to the lungs, liver and brain is frequent.

50. A) Betel nut does not cause carcinoma of urinary bladder.

TUMOURS OF URINARY BLADDER

Risk factors

1. **Chemicals:** Bladder cancer has proven to have occupational basis-affecting workers under sustained exposure to aniline dyes, textiles, leather, paint, organic chemicals and rubber. The provocative agents are 4- aminobiphenyl betanaphthylamine, benzine, and 4-nitrobiphenyl compounds.
2. **Schistosoma haematobium** is also thought to be pathogenetically related to transitional cell carcinoma and squamous cell carcinoma of urinary bladder.
3. **Genetic:** Bladder tumour is associated with mutation of tumour suppressor gene TP 53 with over expression of the T53 protein product.
4. **Smoking:** There is great dealing that the aromatic amines in cigarette smoke (4-aminobiphenyl) and o-toludine are associated with bladder cancer.
5. **Irradiation:** Women who have undergone pelvic radiation therapy for uterine cancer/ cervical cancer have a two to four fold increased risk of developing transitional cell carcinoma of bladder.

6. **Chronic cystitis:** Bladder cancer may be caused by chronic cystitis due to long urinary tract infection, an indwelling catheter or urinary calculi.
7. **Others:** Other sensitizing factors include artificial sweeteners, coffee drinking and phenacetin abuse.

51. D) Causes of bilateral contracted kidneys are:

1. Benign nephrosclerosis
2. Chronic pyelonephritis
3. Chronic glomerulonephritis

52. A) In diabetes kidneys show the appearance of large white kidney.

53. B) Muddy brown casts are pathognomic of acute tubular necrosis. Acute tubular necrosis is a medical condition involving the death of tubular cells that form the tubule.

54. C) Sign and symptoms of chronic renal failure

1. High level of blood urea in the blood, which can result in:

   High blood pressure

   Loss of weight

   Nausea vomiting and diarrhoea which may lead to dehydration

   Headache

   More frequent urination or in greater amounts than usual, with pale urine

   Uraemic pericarditis
2. A build up phosphates in the blood that diseased kidneys cannot filter out may cause:

   Muscle twitches and cramps

   Itching

   Bone damage
3. A build up of potassium in the blood by diseased kidneys cannot filter out may cause:

   Abnormal heart rhythms

   Muscle paralysis
4. Failure to excess fluid may cause:

   Swelling over legs, ankles, feet and face
5. Massive proteinuria

chapter 7

ORAL CAVITY AND SALIVARY GLAND

1. Which of the following malignant salivary gland tumour spreads along the nerves?
   A) Malignant pleomorphic adenoma
   B) Adenoid cystic carcinoma
   C) Mucoepidermoid carcinoma
   D) Acinic cell carcinoma
2. Origin of which of the following tumour is both epithelial as well as mesothelial:
   A) Ameloblastic myxoma
   B) Granular cell ameloblastoma
   C) Ameloblastic fibroma
   D) All of the above
3. The most common tumour of minor and major salivary gland is:
   A) Basal cell adenoma
   B) Sebaceous adenoma
   C) Pleomorphic adenoma
   D) Intraductal adenoma
4. The term used to describe permanent incisors which may be characteristic of congenital syphilis:
   A) Hutchinson's incisors
   B) Blandi's incisors
   C) Turner's incisors
   D) Franklin incisors
5. The most common site for necrotizing sialometaplasia is:
   A) Palate
   B) The buccal mucosa
   C) The lip
   D) The tongue
6. Warthin's tumour can transform into except:
   A) Malignant lymphoma
   B) Adenocarcinoma
   C) Squamous cell carcinoma
   D) Adenoid cystic carcinoma
7. Which of the following type of ameloblastoma has highest propensity towards recurrence?
   A) Follicular type
   B) Granular type
   C) Plexiform type
   D) Acanthomatous type
8. Which of the following condition is known as countryman's lip?
   A) Carcinoma lip
   B) Actinic keratosis lip
   C) Syphilitic ulcer lip
   D) Traumatic ulcer lip
9. Chutta cancer is common in?
   A) Uttar Pradesh
   B) Madhya Pradesh
   C) Andhra Pradesh
   D) Bihar
10. Precancerous intraoral lesion can be responsible for malinancy are except:
    A) Lichen planus
    B) Oral submucus fibrosis
    C) Syphilitic leukoplakia
    D) Hairy leukoplakia

11. Osteoporosis in jaw most probably not related to:
    A) Ovarian agenesis
    B) Hypoandrogenesis
    C) Hyperthyroidism
    D) Adenocarcinoma stomach
12. Warthin's tumour is:
    A) Adenolymphoma parotid
    B) Pleomorphic adenoma
    C) Carcinoma parotid
    D) Carcinoma submandibular
13. Koplik's spots are an early intraoral manifestation of:
    A) Varicella
    B) Variola
    C) Measles
    D) AIDS
14. Most common primary lesion of carcinoma metastasizing to jaws in females?
    A) Breast
    B) Ovarian
    C) Cervix
    D) Gallbladder
15. Pindborg tumour is:
    A) Calcifying epithelial odontogenic tumour
    B) Squamous odontogenic tumour
    C) Ameloblastic fibroma
    D) Ameloblastic fibroadenoma
16. A cyst occurring under the tongue, caused by obstruction of salivary gland is called:
    A) Follicular cyst
    B) Ranula
    C) Dermoid cyst
    D) Dentigerous cyst
17. Following tumours arises from the lining of dentigerous cyst except:
    A) Ameloblastoma
    B) Squamous cell carcinoma
    C) Mucoepidermoid carcinoma
    D) Adenocarcinoma
18. Naevoid basal cell carcinoma syndrome is associated with:
    A) Multiple basal cell carcinoma
    B) Fibrosarcoma
    C) Rhabdomyosarcoma
    D) All of the above
19. Sialolithiasis commonly occurs in:
    A) Sublingual salivary gland
    B) Maxillary sinus
    C) Submandibular salivary gland
    D) Parotid gland
20. Magenta colour tongue and angular cheilitis are as a result of deficiency of which vitamin?
    A) Vitamin B_1
    B) Niacin
    C) Pantothenic acid
    D) Riboflavin
21. Most common site of minor salivary gland tumour is:
    A) Cheek
    B) Palatine
    C) Tonsil
    D) Tongue
22. Papillary cystadenoma lymphomatosum is also called:
    A) Cylindroma
    B) Warthin's tumour
    C) Pleomorphic adenoma
    D) Adenoid cystic carcinoma
23. Biopsy would be of value in the diagnosis of oral lesions of :
    A) Amyloidosis
    B) Carcinoma in situ
    C) Tuberculosis
    D) All of the above
24. The common salivary gland neoplasm that occurs exclusively in parotid gland is:
    A) Pleomorphic adenoma
    B) Warthin's tumour
    C) Ductal papilloma
    D) Mucoepidermoid carcinoma
25. In Warthin's tumour cyst are lined by papillary projections of ___ layered oncocytic epithelium.
    A) Single
    B) Two

C) Tri
D) Many

26. The histogenesis of Pindborg's tumour is from:
A) Cells rests of Malaseez
B) Stratum intermedium
C) Stellate epithelium
D) Dental lamina

27. Most common odontogenic tumour is:
A) Odontoma
B) Ameloblastoma
C) Pindborg's tumour
D) Adenomatoid odontogenic tumour

28. Common variants of ameloblastoma is:
A) Follicular
B) Plexiform
C) Acanthomatous
D) Granular

29. Ranula most commonly involves the:
A) Parotid gland
B) Submandibular gland
C) Sublingual gland
D) Minor salivary gland

30. Ruston bodies are seen in:
A) Rhinoscleroma
B) Odontogenic cysts
C) Megaloblastic anaemia
D) Thalassaemia

31. The untreated dentigenous cyst from its lining may develop all except:
A) Ameloblastoma
B) Epidermoid carcinoma
C) Odontogenic keratocyst
D) Osteomyelitis

32. Which is not true about carcinoma tongue:
A) Commonly adenocarcinoma
B) Lateral border involvement
C) Cervical lymph node involvement
D) Tobacco chewing is a common factor

33. Commonest tumour of jaw is:
A) Ameloblastoma
B) Squamous cell carcinoma
C) Osteosarcoma
D) Osteoma

34. Calculus are most common in ——— salivary gland.
A) Parotid
B) Submandibular
C) Sublingual
D) Accessory

35. Most common precancerous lesion for an oral carcinoma is:
A) Syphilis
B) Leukoplakia
C) Candida patch
D) Traumatic ulcer

36. Magenta coloured tongue is characteristic in deficiencies of:
A) Vitamin A
B) Thiamine deficiency
C) Riboflavin deficiency
D) Intrinsic factor deficiency

37. Amyloid in oral cavity commonly involves:
A) Gingiva
B) Tongue
C) Buccal mucosa
D) Labial mucosa

Answers

1. B) Adenoid cystic carcinoma has a significant propensity for perineural spread and distant metastases.

2. D) Ameloblastic myxoma, ameloblastic fibroma and granular cell ameloblastoma have both epithelial and connective tissue.

3. C) Pleomorphic adenoma is most common parotid gland tumour. It accounts for 70 to 80 percent of all benign parotid tumours. Over 84% of pleomorphic adenomas occur in parotid salivary glands. Intraoral minor salivary gland tumour constitutes approximately 8%.

4. A) Hutchinson's teeth (also known as Hutchinson's incisors) are a sign of congenital syphilis. Babies with this teeth that are smaller and more widely spaced than normal and which have notches on their biting surfaces.

5. A) Necrotising sialometaplasia found mostly on the posterior hard palate, is due to necrosis of minor salivary glands due to trauma (often palatal infiltration of local anaesthetic or trauma during intubation).

6. D) Warthin gave the name papillary cystadenoma lymphomatosum in 1929 in USA. Warthin's tumour is second most common benign lesion in the parotid gland. Very rarely, malignant transformation to lymphoma or adenocarcinoma or squamous cell carcinoma can occur.

7. B) The most common epithelial odontogenic neoplasms of low malignant potential divided into several subtypes including follicular, plexiform, granular cell, desmoplastic, vascular, acanthomatous, papilliferous-keratotic and with dentinoid differentiation. Most characteristics of granular cell ameloblastoma are long duration of tumour, multiple local recurrences, and predominantly in blacks.

8. A) Carcinoma lip is known as Countryman's lip.

9. C) Chutta is a habit that has been strongly associated with the development of cancer of the hard palate. Chutta is a coarsely prepared cheroot that is made by rolling a sundried tobacco leaf into a cylindrical shape that varies from 5 to 9 cm in length. Chutta can be smoked conveniently or in reverse fashion, with the burning end inside the mouth. In India it is common in Andhra Pradesh.

10. D) Precancerous lesions of oral cavity include leukoplakia, erythroplakia, sideropaenic dysphagia, lichen planus, oral submucus fibrosis, discoid lupus erythematosus, actinic keratosis, Plummer-Vinson syndrome, and smokeless tobacco keratosis. Hairy leukoplakia is not a precancerous lesion.

11. D) Causes of osteoporosis of jaw include hyperparathyroidism, hyperprolactinaemia, hyper or hypothyroidism, ovarian or adrenal failure, pituitary tumours, insulin dependent diabetes mellitus and Cushing's syndrome. Neoplastic causes are multiple myeloma and osteolytic metastases.

12. A) Warthin's tumour, also known as papillary cystadenoma lymphomatosum or adenolymphoma, is a benign tumour of salivary gland.

13. C) Koplik spots are pathognomonic for early stage measles.

They are located on the buccal mucosa in the premolar and / molar area. Koplik spots consist of bluish-grey specks against an erythematous background. The lesions are plaque like or nodular and oval or round. If they are numerous, the entire buccal and labial mucosa may give a look of mottled erythema.

14. A) Most common tumour metastasizing in jaw in females is carcinoma breast. Malignant epithelial neoplasms have a tendency to metastasize to bone via the blood stream as well as via lymphatics. Metastatic tumours may present as primary intraoral masses, with or without oral involvement.

In jaws, particularly mandible may be a site of intraosseous metastases.

The lung is the most common site of the primary lesion.

In most site of origin of secondary jaw tumours occur in the following order of frequency: Breast, large intestine, prostate, kidney, thyroid gland, skin (melanoma), endometrium, mesothelioma and testis. Less common sites of origin include the ovary and liver. Chordoma of cervical vertebrae can protrude into the oral cavity.

Metastatic spread occurs more frequently to the mandible than to the maxilla.

15. A) The calcifying epithelial odontogenic tumour, also known as Pindborg tumour or calcifying epithelial tumour first recognized by the Dutch Pathologist Jens Jerger

Pindborg in 1955. Calcifying odontogenic tumour(CEOT) is a rare benign odontogenic neoplasm, forming only 3-4% of all intraosseous odontogenic tumour.

It is odontogenic tumour and thought to arise from the epithelial element of enamel origin. But the exact part from which it originates is not known. However, it has been postulated that it may arise from either the external enamel, stratum intermedium of the enamel organ or from the cellular remnants of the basal sheet or basal stratum of gingival epithelium.

16. B) Renula is a large mucocele arising from the sublingual salivary glands located on the floor of the mouth called glands of Blandin and Nuhn. Renulas may be either mucqus extravasations phenomenon or mucus retention cysts, and most commonly associated with sublingual salivary ducts.

Common cause of renula formation is trauma. Other causes include an obstructed salivary gland or ductal aneurysm. A sarcoid-associated ranula also has been reported.

17. D) This cyst usually associated with non-erupted permanent tooth.

Rarely ameloblastoma and squamous carcinoma, and mucoepidermoid carcinoma have been reported to arise from the cyst lining.

18. D) *'Nevoid basal cell carcinoma'*, is also known as *'Goltiz's'* tumour or Gorlin tumour. It is a condition inherited as an autosomal dominant trait and characterized by a predisposition for keratocystic odontogenic tumour (Odontogenic keratocysts) and skin cancers, especially basal cell carcinoma, as well as the presence of a number of abnormalities of tumours in the skeletal, nervous, endocrine and other systems. Recent work in molecular genetics has shown NBCCs to be caused by mutations in the PTCH (patched) gene found on chromosome arm 9q.

Other tumours, including fibrosarcoma, rhabdomyosarcoma, and meningioma may be increased in frequency in persons with NBCC syndrome.

19. C) Salivary calculi are almost exclusively located in the major salivary glands.

They are common in submandibular gland (Wharton's duct), sublingual and minor salivary gland. It is uncommon in parotid gland (Stensen's duct). Sublingual gland is affected in 2% of cases and minor salivary glands in another 2%. High frequency of submandibular involvement is believed to be secondary to the tortuous course of Wharton's duct, high levels of calcium and phosphate, and the relative dependent position of the glands thus facilitating stasis and stone formation.

20. D) In riboflavin deficiency oral mucosa is pale due to anaemia.

Lips: Redness, and shiny appearance of lips is due to desquamation of epithelium.

Cheilosis: Lesions at the mucocutaneous junction at the angle of the mouth leading to painful fissures.

Tongue: Painful glossitis, tongue assuming a red purple (magenta) colour. There is complete atrophy of papillae gives rise to smooth and glazed tongue.

21. B) Intraoral minor salivary gland tumour constitutes approximately 8%. The palatal glands are the most affected in this group (65-75%). Other sites included in oral cavity are sublingual glands, cheek, and floor of the mouth.

22. B) Papillary cystadenoma lymphomatosum is also known as Warthin's tumour.

23. D) Biopsy would be of value in the diagnosis of amyloidosis of tongue, carcinoma in situ, malignant tumours of oral cavity, tuberculosis of larynx.

24. B) Although pleomorphic adenoma is more common Warthin's tumour is almost exclusive to parotid gland.

25. B) The inner layer cells are tall columnar with

a finely granular and eosinophilic cytoplasm and outer layer cells are oncocytic and triangular.

26. C) It is odontogenic tumour and thought to arise from the epithelial element of enamel origin. But the exact part from which it originates is not known. However, it has been postulated that it may arise from either the external enamel, stratum intermedium of the enamel organ or from the cellular remnants of the basal sheet or basal stratum of gingival epithelium.

27. B) Most common odontogenic tumour is ameloblastoma.

28. A) Follicular ameloblastoma is the most common histological type (65%) followed by plexiform ameloblastoma (13%), desmoplastic ameloblastoma (5%), basal cell (3%) and acanthomatous (4%).

29. C) Ranula is a large mucocele arising from the sublingual salivary glands located on the floor of the mouth called glands of Blandin and Nuhn. Ranulas may be either mucous extravasations phenomenon or mucus retention cysts, and most commonly associated with sublingual salivary ducts.

30. B) Ruston bodies are linear or curved hyaline bodies presumably of haematogenous origin found in the epithelial lining of odontogenic cysts.

31. D) This cyst usually associated with non-erupted permanent tooth.

Rarely ameloblastoma and squamous carcinoma, and mucoepidermoid carcinoma and odontogenic keratocyst have been reported to arise from the cyst lining.

32. A) Microscopically, the majority of carcinomas arising at front of tongue are squamous cell tumours of varying degrees of cornification and differentiation. Some invasive cancers are well-differentiated variants; others show undifferentiated and an occasional carcinoma consists of predominantly of clear cells filled with glycogen. A painful non-healing ulcer is usually present on the lateral surface of tongue. Spread through lymphatics is early. The spread takes place into submental and submaxillary lymph nodes, superior and inferior deep cervical nodes and even to the supraclavicular nodes. The tumours of the posterior third-the upper deep cervical group of lymph nodes of both the sides of the neck may be involved. Excessive use of tobacco, taken as snuff, chewed, smoked in pipes or as cigars or cigarettes have been implicated as predisposing agents.

33. A) Most common tumour of jaw is ameloblastoma.

34. B) Salivary calculi are almost exclusively located in the major salivary glands.

They are common in submandibular gland (Wharton's duct), sublingual and minor salivary gland. It is uncommon in parotid gland (Stensen's duct). Sublingual gland is affected in 2% of cases and minor salivary glands in another 2%. High frequency of submandibular involvement is believed to be secondary to the tortuous course of Wharton's duct, high levels of calcium and phosphate, and the relative dependent position of the glands thus facilitating stasis and stone formation.

35. B) Most common precancerous lesion for an oral carcinoma is leukoplakia. Precancerous lesions of oral cavity include leukoplakia, erythroplakia, sideropaenic dysphagia, lichen planus, oral submucus fibrosis, discoid lupus erythematosus, actinic keratosis, Plummer-Vinson syndrome, and smokeless tobacco keratosis.

36. C) Magenta coloured tongue is seen in patients with riboflavin deficiency.

37. B) Most common oral manifestation of amyloidosis is macroglossia which occurs in 20% of patients.

chapter 8

HEPATOBILIARY PATHOLOGY

1. Association of carcinoma gallbladder with gall stones is:
   A) 20%
   B) 50%
   C) 80%
   D) 90%
2. Gallbladder is capable of distending how many ml bile?
   A) 50 ml
   B) 40 ml
   C) 30 ml
   D) 20 ml
3. Parasite causes cirrhosis is:
   A) E. histiolytica
   B) Schistosoma haematobium
   C) Taenia echinococcus
   D) Wucheria bancrofti.
4. Inherited diseases causes cirrhosis except:
   A) Wilson's disease
   B) Alpha-1 antitrypsin deficiency
   C) Haemochromatosis
   D) Biliary cirrhosis
5. Conjugated hyperbilirubinaemia is seen in:
   A) Gilbert's disease
   B) Criggler Najjar syndrome
   C) Breast milk syndrome
   D) Dubin Jonhson's syndrome
6. Which of these diseases is an autoimmune disease most commonly found in young men?
   A) Primary biliary cirrhosis
   B) Primary sclerosing cholangitis
   C) Autoimmune hepatitis
   D) Alpha-1 antitrypsin deficiency
7. Which of the following structures does not form portal triad:
   A) Portal vein
   B) Hepatic artery
   C) Hepatic vein
   D) Bile duct
8. Which is not a paraneoplastic sydrome of hepatocellular carcinoma:
   A) Hypercalcaemia
   B) Hypoglycaemia
   C) Erythrocytosis
   D) Hyperglycaemia
9. Normal weight of liver is
   A) 900 gram
   B) 1000 gram
   C) 1400 gram
   D) 2000 gram
10. Which of the following has weakest association with HCC:
    A) Hepatitis C
    B) Hepatitis B
    C) Oral contraceptives
    D) Smoking
11. Indirect bilirubin is increased in except:
    A) Erythroblastosis fetalis
    B) Criggler Najjar syndrome

C) Rotor syndrome
D) Gilbert's disease

12. Which of these diseases are associated with anti-mitochondrial antibody?
A) Primary biliary cirrhosis
B) Primary sclerosing cholangitis
C) Autoimmune hepatitis
D) Hepatitis B carrier state

13. A child with acute liver failure, the most important prognostic factor for death is:
A) Increasing transaminases
B) Increasing bilirubin
C) Increasing prothrombin time
D) Gram-negative sepsis

14. Which is not true regarding haemangioendothelioma of liver:
A) It is a rare tumour
B) It is highly vascular
C) It involves both lobes of liver
D) In 50% of cases it has extrahepatic spread.

15. Mid-zonal necrosis occurs in:
A) Toxaemia of pregnancy
B) Infective hepatitis
C) Yellow fever
D) Chronic venous congestion

16. An important physical signs of portal hypertension in a patient of cirrhosis of liver is:
A) Gynaecomastia
B) Hepatomegaly
C) Palmar erythemia
D) Splenomegaly

17. Lead pipe cirrhosis of liver seen in infestation by:
A) Plasmodium
B) Schistosoma
C) Fasciola hepatica
D) Clonorchis sinensis

18. In a patient with high-grade fever, rigors, and tender hepatomegaly, the most likely diagnosis is:
A) Carcinoma of liver
B) Liver abscess
C) Malaria
D) Heart failure

19. Anchovy sauce aspirate is characteristic of which of the following:
A) Hydatid cyst
B) Amoebic abscess liver
C) Malaria
D) Pyaemic abscess of liver

20. Mallory hyaline are seen in:
A) Alcoholic hepatitis
B) Wilson's disease
C) Primary biliary cirrhosis
D) All of the above

21. Ascitis in portal cirrhosis is due to:
A) Portal hypertension
B) Hypoproteinaemia
C) Sodium retention
D) All of the above.

22. Dubin Johnson's syndrome test used is:
A) Gamma Glutamyl transaminase
B) Liver biopsy
C) Hippuric acid test
D) Transaminases

23. Best test for liver function is:
A) Alanine aminotransferase
B) Serum bilirubin
C) Prothrombin time
D) Serum albumin

24. Mallory body in hepatic cells in alcoholic liver disease is type of:
A) Thin actin filament
B) Thick myosin filament
C) Microtubule
D) Intermediate filament

25. The progression to cirrhosis is seen in:
A) Chronic persistent hepatitis
B) Chronic lobular hepatitis
C) Chronic active hepatitis
D) All of the above

26. Earliest symptoms of biliary cirrhosis is:
A) Jaundice
B) Pale stools
C) Pruritis
D) Hepatomegaly

27. Stain used for demonstration of HbsAg in liver cells is:
   A) Haematoxylin and Eosin
   B) Orcein stain
   C) Giemsa stain
   D) PAS stain
28. Following are the primary malignancies which show occult malignancy in liver except:
   A) Carcinoma stomach
   B) Carcinoma breast
   C) Central nervous system tumours
   D) Carcinoma lung
29. Which of the following is not likely to cause large bile duct obstruction:
   A) Hodgkin's lymphoma at the liver hilum
   B) Primary biliary cirrhosis
   C) Gall stones
   D) Carcinoma of head of pancreas
30. Following are characteristics of chronic active hepatitis except:
   A) Piece meal necrosis
   B) Lobular hepatitis
   C) Portal inflammation
   D) Does not progress to cirrhosis
31. Which of the following component is an indicator of post infection and subsequent immunity to hepatitis B-viral infection?
   A) HbsAG
   B) ABcAg
   C) HbeAg
   D) Anti Hbs
32. Councilman bodies are seen in:
   A) Viral hepatitis
   B) Cirrhosis of liver
   C) Chronic active hepatitis
   D) Carcinoma of liver
33. Prognostic features of chronic alcoholism is;
   A) Fatty infiltration
   B) Portal fibrosis
   C) Liver cirrhosis
   D) Central hyaline sclerosis
34. The most common association seen with carcinoma gall bladder is:
   A) Cystic node involvement
   B) Secondaries liver
   C) Duodenal infiltration
   D) Peritoneal deposits
35. Most common cause of pyogenic liver abscess is:
   A) Cryptogenic
   B) Ascending cholangitis
   C) Portal pyaemia
   D) Haematogenous
36. First human liver transplantation was performed by:
   A) Thomas Starzl
   B) Alexis Carnel
   C) Christian Bernard
   D) Halstead
37. Unconjugated bilirubinaemia is seen in all except:
   A) Rotor syndrome
   B) Thalassaemia
   C) G6PD deficiency
   D) Criggler-Najjar syndrome
38. Unconjugated hyperbilirubinaemia is found in A/E
   A) Sclerosing cholangitis
   B) Haematoma
   C) Thalassaemia
   D) Prolong breast milk feeding
39. Specific tumour marker of hepatoblastoma is:
   A) CEA (carcino embryonic antigen)
   B) Alpha feto protein
   C) CA-125
   D) Lactic dehydrogenase
40. Hydatid cyst occurs most commonly in:
   A) Liver
   B) Lungs
   C) Brain
   D) Spleen

41. Acute infection with HBV is characterized by:
A) HbsAg
B) Anti HbsAg
C) IgM anti HbcAg and HbsAg
D) Anti HBeAg

42. Extrahepatic complications of hepatitis B virus infection:
A) Polyarteritis nodosa
B) Membranous or mesangioproliferative glomerulonephritis
C) Erythema nodosum
D) All of the above

43. Hepar lobatum is due to:
A) Hepatitis A
B) Syphilis
C) Alcoholic cirrhosis
D) Hydatid cyst

44. Piecemeal necrosis is seen in:
A) Alcoholic cirrhosis
B) Biliary cirrhosis
C) Chronic active hepatitis
D) Indian childhood cirrhosis

45. Alkaline phosphatase is increased beyond 30 KA units in:
A) Obstructive jaundice
B) Hypothyroidism
C) Leukaemia
D) Polycythaemia vera

46. Central necrosis of liver is seen in:
A) CCF
B) Yellow fever
C) Phosphorus poisoning
D) Carbon tetrachloride

47. Bridging necrosis is seen in:
A) Chronic active hepatitis
B) Typhoid fever
C) Yellow fever
D) Alcoholic liver disease

48. True about physiological jaundice:
A) Direct bilirubin increase
B) Appears within 24 hours
C) More severe in premature
D) None

49. Commonest cause of jaundice within 6 hours of birth.
A) Breast milk jaundice
B) Physiological jaundice
C) Biliary atresia
D) Rh incompatibility

50. Charcot's triad is seen in:
A) Acute pancreatitis
B) Haemophilia
C) Stone in bile duct
D) Chronic cholecystitis

51. Strawberry gallbladder is seen in:
A) Gangrene of gall bladder
B) Procelain gall bladder
C) Adenomatosis
D) Cholesterolosis

52. Klastskin tumour is:
A) At the junction of cystic duct and bile duct
B) At bile duct
C) At ampulla of Vater
D) At the junction of bile duct

53. All of the following are indications of liver transplantation except:
A) Hepatocellular carcinoma
B) Cirrhosis
C) Alcoholic hepatitis
D) Biliary atresia

54. Marker of hepatitis B in the window period is:
A) HbsAg
B) Anti-HbsAg
C) Anti-Hbc
D) HbeAg

Answers

1. C) Association of carcinoma with gallstones is 80%. Chronic irritation caused by gall bladder stones can leads to proliferation, metaplasia, dysplasia, and carcinoma.

2. A) Gallbladder is capable of distending 50 ml of bile.

3. B) Deposition of eggs of Schistosoma mansoni is followed by the formation of granulomata and the development of portal fibrosis. Ova produce granulomas in the acute phase followed by pipe stem fibrosis in chronic phase.

4. D) Inherited diseases causing cirrhosis include: Wilson's disease, haemochromatosis, alpha-1 antitrypsin deficiency, cystic fibrosis, galactosemia, and glycogen storage diseases.

5. D) Conjugated hyperbilirubinaemia is seen in Dubin Johnson's syndrome. Dubin–Johnson syndrome is a chronic, benign, intermittent jaundice with conjugated hyperbilirubinaemia and with hyperbilirubinuria. It is autosomal recessive and is most frequent in the Middle East among Iranian Jews. The mutation responsible is in the gene encoding CMOAT (Multi specific) organic anion transporter.

6. B) Primary sclerosing cholangitis is characterized by progressive inflammation, and fibrosis of intrahepatic bile ducts. It predominantly affects young men with inflammatory bowel disease.

7. C) Hepatic vein does not form part of the portal triad. It forms the central vein around which hepatocytes are arranged and on the periphery is the portal triad consisting of portal vein posteriorly, the bile duct on the right, and hepatic artery on the left.

8. D) Less than 1% of hepatocellular carcinoma present as a paraneoplastic syndrome most commonly hypercalcaemia, hypoglycaemia, and erythrocytosis.

9. C) Normal weight of liver varies from 1200 gram to 1400 gram.

10. C) Several cases of liver cell carcinomas, either alone or in association liver cell adenomas have been reported in women taking contraceptive pills.

11. C) Rotor syndrome is a rare, relatively benign autosomal recessive bilirubin disorder of unknown origin. The liver cells are not pigmented. The main symptom is a non-itching jaundice. There is a rise in bilirubin in the patient's serum mainly of the conjugated type. In Criggler-Najjar syndrome, Gilbert's disease, and erythroblastosis foetalis unconjugated bilirubin is increased.

12. A) Antimitochondrial antibody (AMA) is detected in 90% of people with primary biliary cirrhosis.

13. C) In patients with acute liver failure the prognostic factor is prolong prothrombin time. The prothrombin time, which is also called protime or PT, is a test that is used to assess blood clotting. When liver is significantly injured, these proteins are not normally produced. There is severe bleeding and death.

14. D) Haemangioendothelioma is a rare neoplasm of vascular origin that involves both hepatic lobes. In 27 to 30% of patients have extrahepatic metastases at the time of diagnosis.

15. C) Mid zonal necrosis of liver occurs in yellow fever. Periportal necrosis occurs in toxaemia of pregnancy. In cases of chronic venous congestion liver there is centrivenular necrosis of liver cells. In cases of hepatitis necrosis may occur in single liver cells, focal necrosis, bridging or massive necrosis.

16. D) One of the most common finding in portal hypertension is splenomegaly. The spleen is enlarged from normal 300 grams or less between 500 grams to 1000 grams.

17. B) Schistosoma mansoni is common in Egypt and other parts of Africa. Schistosoma Japonica is found in China, Japan and the Philippines. Both infections involve the liver. Deposition of eggs is followed by the formation of granulomata and the development of portal fibrosis. Granulomas are composed of macrophages, eosinophils, epitheloid cells and giant cells around the ovum. The ova produce granulomas in the acute phase followed by pipe stem fibrosis in chronic phase.

18. B) In this case patient have fever and rigors. This indicates that patient has acute infection. Since liver is tender and enlarged there is suspicion of abscess liver. In cases of carcinoma liver and malaria there is no liver tenderness. In congestion, liver is tender but there is no history of fever with rigors.

19. B) Amoebic liver abscesses are common in upper quadrant of right lobe of liver in the posterosuperior portion than left lobe. This is explained by the streamline phenomenon of the portal venous supply. More often an abscess is more than 10 cm in size. The wall of an abscess has an irregular shaggy pale peripheral necrotic rim and fibrous tissue. The wall consists of compressed liver tissue. Central portion is filled by thick reddish brown fluid **anchovy sauce or chocolate sauce** composed of necrotic liver cell debris fibrin and blood.

20. D) Mallory hyaline are classically found in liver of people suffering from alcoholic liver disease, alcoholic hepatitis, alcoholic cirrhosis, Wilson's disease, Primary biliary cirrhosis, and hepatocellular carcinoma.

21. D) Ascitis in active portal hypertension is due to hypoalbuminaemia, portal hypertension, post-sinusoidal block, inferior vena cava hypertension, hyperaldosteronism, and splanchnic vasodilatation.

22. B) Conjugated hyperbilirubinaemia is seen in Dubin Johnson's syndrome. Dubin–Johnson syndrome is a chronic, benign, intermittent jaundice with conjugated hyperbiliru-binaemia and with hyperbilirubinuria. It is an autosomal recessive disease. In cases of Dubin-Johnson disease GGT, transaminases and Hippuric acid test is normal. Dubin Johnson syndrome is usually diagnosed by liver biopsy, the liver is deeply pigmented as a result of an intracellular melanin-like substance but otherwise normal.

23. A) Alanine aminotransferase is an enzyme mainly found in the liver. It is increased in serum in early liver damage. It is the best test for detecting hepatitis. Serum bilirubin, prothrombin time and serum albumin are affected in liver diseases other than liver cell necrosis.

24. D) Mallory body is called after the American pathologist who described it in 1911. Mallory bodies are abnormal aggregates of cellular intermediate filament proteins are present as eosinophilic hyaline in hepatocytes in cases of alcoholic hepatitis.

25. C) Chronic active hepatitis progresses to cirrhosis. Chronic persistent hepatitis and lobular hepatitis does not progress to cirrhosis. Chronic hepatitis may be defined as inflammation of liver continuing without improvement for at least six months.

26. C) Pruritis is earliest symptom of biliary cirrhosis. Bile acids in the serum and tissues leads to intense generalized itching. No bile passes into the intestine, and stools are clay coloured. Liver is enlarged and nodular jaundice is obstructive type with increase level of conjugated bilirubin.

27. B) Orcein stain. The HbsAg (hepatitis surface antigen) occurs most frequently as cytoplasmic inclusions in hepatocytes. Kupffer cell cytoplasm may also show the antigen. If many hepatocytes are affected, the antigen appears as fine granules either diffusely spread throughout the cytoplasm or concentrated in the cytoplasm peripheral to the sinusoid space. This is called the ground glass appearance. In single cell involvement, the HbsAg appears as oval, round or irregularly shaped aggregates in the cytoplasm, especially in the perinuclear region.

28. C) Occult malignancies in liver are from carcinoma stomach, colon, breast, pancreas, and bronchus. Central nervous system tumours are highly malignant but never metastasize.

29. B) Primary biliary cirrhosis causes intrahepatic obstruction.

Causes of extrahepatic bile duct obstruction:

- Gall stone obstruction of biliary tree
- Carcinoma head of pancreas, extrahepatic bile ducts and ampulla of Vater
- Extrahepatic biliary atresia
- Biliary stricture and choledochal cysts
- Primary sclerosing cholangitis (extrahepatic)
- Liver flukes
- Ascaris lumbricoides
- Pressure from outside by enlarged lymph nodes at porta hepatis

30. D) Characteristics of chronic active hepatitis are:

1. Piece meal necrosis
2. Lobular necrosis
3. Bridging necrosis
4. Portal inflammation
5. Progression to cirrhosis

31. D) Hepatitis B surface antibody (anti HBs) produced in response to HBV surface antigen, levels in the blood rise during the recovery phase.

Anti HBs test is used to detect previous exposure to HBV, can also be acquired from successful vaccination. This test is more to determine the need for vaccination (if anti HBs) is absent or to determine if a person has recovered from infections and is immune (cannot get the infection again).

32. A) In viral hepatitis, single liver cells, which die one by one (necrobiosis and apoptosis). Single liver cells may also undergo acidophilic or eosinophilic necrosis. The cells are eosinophilic granular with pyknotic nucleus extruded leaving the acidophilic or Councilman bodies.

33. C) Alcoholism causes development of large fatty globules throughout the liver and can begin to occur after a few days of heavy drinking. Cirrhosis is a late stage of serious liver disease marked by inflammation, and fibrosis.

34. B) By the time gallbladder cancers are discovered most have invaded the liver directly, and many have extended to cystic duct and adjacent bile ducts and porta hepatic lymph nodes. The peritoneum, gastrointestinal tract and lungs are less common sites of seedling.

35. B) In western word, bacterial and fungal abscesses are more common, representing a complication of an infection elsewhere. The organisms reach the liver through following pathways:

1. Ascending infection in the biliary tract (ascending cholangitis)
2. Vascular seeding, either portal or arterial
3. Direct invasion of the liver from a nearby source
4. Penetrating injury

Pyogenic (bacterial) hepatic abscesses may occur as solitary or multiple lesions, ranging from millimeters to massive lesions many centimeters in diameters.

Bacteraemic spread through the arterial or portal systems tends to produce multiple small abscesses, where as direct extension and trauma usually cause solitary large abscess. Biliary abscesses, which are usually multiple may contain purulent material in adjacent bile ducts.

36. A) The first human liver transplant was performed in 1963 by a surgical team led by Dr Thomas Starzl of Denver, Colorado, United State.

37. A) Rotor syndrome is a rare, relatively benign autosomal recessive disorder of unknown origin. It causes increase in conjugated bilirubin. In rotor syndrome liver cells are not pigmented. In cases of thalassaemia, G6PD deficiency and Criggler-Najjar syndrome there is increase in unconjugated bilirubin.

38. A) PRIMARY SCLEROSING CHOLANGITIS (PSC) is a chronic autoimmune cholestatic liver disease that causes bile duct inflammation. PSC often accompanies other autoimmune disorders. The disease shows a male preponderance of 3:1 and in 70% of cases associated with chronic inflammatory bowel disease, especially ulcerative colitis. It predominantly affects young men. Inflammatory and fibrosing process narrows and eventually obstructs the intrahepatic and extrahepatic bile ducts.

Primary sclerosing cholangitis is characterized by progressive inflammation, destruction and fibrosis of intrahepatic and extrahepatic bile ducts.

Retrograde cholangiography shows diagnostic changes in the extrahepatic ducts. Strictures and outpouring can give a beaded appearance. Inflammation of bile ducts leads to concentric ' onion-skin' fibrosis.

Investigations

Cojugated bilirubin is increased.

- Perinuclear antineutrophil cytoplasmic antibody (PNACA) has been reported in 26% to 85% of primary sclerosing cholangitis subjects and 75% of ulcerative colitis with PSC.
- An increased prevalence of HLA-A1-B8, and DR 3 alleles in PSC have been described but remain nonspecific.
- Alkaline phosphatase values often predominate with elevation up to three times the upper limit of normal in nearly 95% of cases.
- Serum alanine as asparate transaminase levels can also be found between two and three times the upper limit of normal.
- Serum immunoglobulin levels and autoantibodies are associated with primary sclerosing cholangitis. Elevations in IgG and IgM is up to 40% and 60% of individuals are observed.
- Antinuclear antibodies and smooth muscle antibody (ASMs) can also be detected. Antimitochondrial antibodies (AMAs) are exceedingly rare in PSC.

In cases of hepatoma, Thalassaemia, and prolong breast milk feeding there is increased unconjugated bilirubin

39. B) The alpha fetoprotein is also used as a tumour marker for cancer such as hepatoblastoma. In a normal human, the AFP level is usually under 10, in children with hepatoblastoma the number can be much higher.

Hepatoblastoma often produces a protein which can be detected in the blood. Levels of alpha fetoprotein (AFP) can be used as way to determine whether the tumour is responding to treatment (AFP level is decreased), whether there is no evidence of disease or if there is an indication of relapse (increased levels of AFP).

40. A) Hydatid cyst primarily affects the liver (70 % to 93%). The second most common organ involved is the lung (5 to 15%). Other sites include: Spleen, brain, heart, kidneys, and female genital tract.

This is caused by Ecchinococcus granulosis. Man is the intermediate host. After ingestion, the egg loses its membrane and liberated hexacanth embryo penetrates into the intestinal wall through portal vein it is carried to liver where they produce hydatid cysts or hollow bladder. Right lobe of liver is usually affected. Cyst is unilocular and it grows slowly 1cm per month. Cyst grows slowly 1-5cm in diameter by 6 months and final size of 5 to 20cm in one year.

CLINICAL FEATURES

Uncomplicated hydatid cyst may be silent. Clinical manifestations occur when cyst reaches about 10 cm diameter and palpable when it reaches 20 cm. It may produce dull ache in the liver area and abdominal distention. There is hepatomegaly. Major clinical manifestations are caused by mechanical compression of the surrounding tissue. They include jaundice, cholangitis, reactive hepatitis, and cirrhosis of liver and portal hypertension.

Rupture of cyst: Cyst ruptures spontaneously or through trauma or surgery. When a cyst ruptures into bile duct or gall bladder, clinical symptoms may mimic those of choledocholithiasis, cholangitis, and cholecystitis. Contents of cyst may be expelled into the peritoneal cavity; pleural cavity, pulmonary parenchyma or bronchi, pericardial cavity, renal pelvis or intestine may be involved. The most dangerous complication is sudden rupture of a cyst into blood vessel that may lead to anaphylactic reaction with dyspnoea, asthma, pruritis and cyanosis. In suspected cases of cyst in liver, needle biopsy should not be attempted.

Diagnosis

1. **Radiological and ultrasound examination**
2. Eosinophilia
3. Casoni's test

41. C) The hepatitis B surface antigen (HbsAg) is most frequently used to screen for the presence of this infection. It is the first detectable viral antigen to appear during infection. However, early in an infection this antigen may not be present and it may be undectable later in the infection as it is being cleared by the body. The infectious virion contains an "inner core particle" enclosing viral genome. The icosohedral core particle is made of 180 or 240 copies of core proteins alternatively known as hepatitis B core antigen or HbcAg. During the 'window' in which the host remains infected but is successfully clearing the virus, IgM antibodies to hepatitis B core antigen (anti Hbc IgM may be only serological evidence of disease. Therefore most hepatitis B diagnostic panels contain HbsAg and total anti Hbc (both IgM and IgG).

42. D) Extrahepatic manifestations of hepatitis B infection include:

- Polyarteritis nodosa
- Membranous or membranoproliferative glomerulonephritis
- Leucocytoclastic vasculitis
- Arthritis and acute serum sickness
- Erythema nodosum
- Raynaud's phenomenon
- Mononeuritis multiplex
- LGB syndrome
- Pericarditis
- Pancreatitis

43. B) Hepar lobatum term generally refers to liver abnormalities in tertiary syphilis. In some instances, chemotherapy for metastatic liver cancer (especially from the breast) can lead to similar changes.

The liver shows a lobulated contour with capsular indentations from which fibrous septa extend deep into the parenchyma.

The fibrous septa can surround the degenerated centre of tumour nodules and may contain macrophages and residual tumour.

Typical features of cirrhosis such as regenerated nodules are not observed.

44. C) Hallmark of chronic active hepatitis is piecemeal necrosis, in which the cells at the border between the connective tissue of portal system and the hepatocytes are destroyed. This necrosis leads to cirrhosis and liver failure.

Chronic active hepatitis is caused by many factors including hepatitis B, C, or D virus, autoimmunity, and idiosyncratic drug preparations.

All of these causes can lead to the inflammation of the liver, especially around the portal veins.

45. A) A striking increase > 30 units occur in extrabiliary obsctruction, intrahepatic cholestasis and primary biliary cirrhosis. Alkaline phosphatase (ALP) is an enzyme in the cells lining biliary ducts of liver. ALP levels in plasma will rise with large bile duct obstruction, intrahepatic cholestasis, or infiltrative diseases of liver.

Possible causes of increased levels of plasma alkaline phosphatase include:

I. Hepatobiliary disease including cholestasis:
   - Cholestasis: Increased serum alkaline phosphatase in extrahepatic cholestasis is due to
     1. Much increased in hepatic synthesis
     2. Much decreased in biliary excretion
   - Hepatocyte disease: Such as viral hepatitis which cause moderate elevations in ALP.

II. **Bone diseases:** Bone isoenzyme of alkaline phosphatase, reflecting increased osteoblastic activity, it may be raised in:
   - Paget's disease
   - Osteomalacia and rickets
   - Renal osteodystrophy
   - Bone metastasis (breast cancer)
   - Primary bone tumours e.g., sarcoma
   - Recent fracture

III. Growing child

IV. During pregnancy the placenta secretes its own isoenzyme, which raises total alkaline phosphatase concentration.

V. Malignancies resulting in expression of ALP-like gene e.g., seminomas.

Normal level of serum alkaline phosphatase 3 to 13 units/100ml (King and Armstrong)

46. A) CCF

Different types of liver cell necrosis

LIVER CELL NECROSIS

1. **Single scattered** liver cells, which die one by one (necrobiosis or apoptosis). Single liver cells may also undergo acidophilic or eosinophilic necrosis. The cells are eosinophilic granular with pyknotic nucleus extruded leaving the acidophilic or **councilman body.**
2. **Lytic necrosis**: Hepatocytes may osmotically swell and rupture.
3. **Focal necrosis**: Necrosis of small group of hepatocytes seen in severe toxemia, drug induced hepatitis, diphtheria, typhoid and scarlet fever.
4. **Confluent necrosis**: Necrosis of large group of hepatocytes seen in severe viral hepatitis, drug induced and acute ischemic liver injury.
5. **Bridging necrosis**: Confluent necrosis may extend between contiguous hepatic venules or hepatic venules and portal tract.
6. **Massive necrosis**: Diffuse necrosis in which cells in a number of lobules are affected, seen in acute yellow atrophy of liver, infective hepatitis, phosphorus, lead, arsenic, chloroform, carbon tetrachloride poisoning.

Zonal necrosis in which the cells in certain zones of liver lobules are affected, it may be:

1. Perivenular or centrilobular necrosis
   Necrosis of liver cells around central vein due to drugs and toxins e.g., alcohol and paracetamol and congestive cardiac failure
2. **Mid-zonal necrosis** seen in yellow fever and streptococcal infection.
3. **Periportal zonal necrosis is** seen in eclampsia.

Piece meal necrosis is defined as destruction of liver cells at an interface between parenchyma and connective tissue.

Submassive necrosis: Necrosis of entire lobule occurs.

47. A) Bridging necrosis: Confluent necrosis may extend between contiguous hepatic venules or hepatic venules and portal tract. It is characteristically seen in chronic active hepatitis.

48. C) Physiological jaundice: Occurring in more than 50% of newborns. This jaundice is due to the immaturity of the baby's liver, which leads to a slow processing of bilirubin. It is due to relative deficiency of glucoronyl transferase and deficient protein ligandin in the neonatal liver. Occasionally neonatal hypothyroidism manifests as prolonged physiological jaundice because UGT levels are lower than normal. If high levels of jaundice do not clear up, phototherapy is choice of treatment.

Indirect bilirubin is increased. It generally appears at 2 to 4 days of age and disappears by 1 to 2 weeks of age.

49. D) Commonest cause of jaundice within 6 hours of birth is Rh incompatibility.

Physiological icterus usually appears on 3rd and regress by 7th day.

Breast milk jaundice starts on 4 to 7 days and normally lasts from 3 to 10 weeks.

Jaundice in cases of biliary atresia occurs at birth.

50. D) Charcot's cholangitis triad is the combination of jaundice, fever usually with rigors and right upper quadrant abdominal pain. It occurs as a result of ascending cholangitis (an infection of the bile duct in the liver).

51. D) Strawberry gallbladder is also known as cholesterolosis or lipoidosis of gallbladder, is a change in gallbladder wall due to excess cholesterol. The name strawberry gallbladder comes from the typically stippled appearance of the mucosal surface on gross examination, which resembles the appearance of a strawberry.

52. D) Klastskin tumour develops in cells that line the bile ducts in the liver where the right and left ducts meet. It is a type of cholangiocarcinoma.

53. C) Common indications of liver transplant

- Cholestatic disease: Primary biliary cirrhosis, sclerosing cholangitis, secondary biliary cirrhosis, biliary atresia, cystic fibrosis.
- Chronic hepatitis: Hepatitis B, Hepatitis C, hepatitis D, autoimmune chronic hepatitis, cryptogenic cirrhosis, chronic drug toxicity or toxin exposure.
- Alcoholic cirrhosis
- Metabolic diseases
  - Wilson's disease
  - Alpha-1-antitrypsin deficiency
  - Glycogen storage disease
  - Tyrosinaemia
  - Familial amyloidotic polyneuropathy
- Primary hepatic tumours—Hepatocellular carcinoma

Contraindications

- HIV infection
- Active alcohol or substance abuse
- Systemic infections
- Life limiting-co-existing medical conditions: Advanced heart, lung or neurologic conditions
- Active septic infections

54. C) During the window period (or equivalence zone) of hepatitis B, both serological markers HbsAg (hepatitis B surface antigen) and Anti-HBs (antibody against HbsAg) are negative (which is due to the fact that, although there are anti-Hbs antibodies present they are actively bound to the HbsAG). Other serological markers, IgM (antibody) against HBc can be positive at this point.

chapter 9

GASTROINTESTINAL TRACT

1. All are features of Plummer-Vinson syndrome except:
   A) Oesophageal web
   B) Iron deficiency
   C) Achalasia cardia
   D) Dysphagia
2. Oesophageal cancer is commonly associated with?
   A) Alcohol abuse
   B) Achalasia
   C) Reflux
   D) Smoking
3. A 60-year-old patient with pernicious anaemia, the stomach exhibit one of the following characteristically:
   A) Increased number of argentaffin cells
   B) Hyperacidity
   C) Mucosal atrophy
   D) H. pylori infection
4. Which of the following circulating antibodies has the best sensitivity a specificity for the diagnosis of celiac disease:
   A) Anti-endomysial antibody
   B) Anti-tissue transglutaminase antibody
   C) Anti-gliadin antibody
   D) Anti-reticulin antibody
5. Which of the following conditions is thought to be not associated H. pylori infection
   A) Gastric carcinoma
   B) MALTOMA
   C) Barrett's oesophagitis
   D) Pernicious anaemia
6. Commonest site of occurrence of carcinoid in the gastrointestinal tract is:
   A) Stomach
   B) Appendix
   C) Sigmoid colon
   D) Jejunum
7. All of the following are likely complication of duodenal ulcers except:
   A) Haemorrhage
   B) Perforation
   C) Scarring with obstruction
   D) Malignant change
8. Most common cause of gastric outlet obstruction in India is:
   A) Tuberculosis
   B) Cancer of stomach
   C) Duodenal lymphoma
   D) Peptic ulcer disease
9. Carcinoma of which organ causes pseudomyxoma peritonei.
   A) Testis
   B) Lung
   C) Liver
   D) Appendix
10. Dysphagia can be associated with each of the following except:
    A) Myasthenia gravis
    B) Iron deficiency anaemia
    C) Parkinsonism
    D) Oesophageal varices

11. Most common site for oesophageal carcinoma is:
   A) Upper third
   B) Middle third
   C) Lower third
   D) Postcricoid region
12. Hour glass deformity of stomach is seen in:
   A) Gastric ulcer
   B) Gastric carcinoma
   C) Gastric lymphoma
   D) Corrosive stricture
13. True about Hirschprung's disease
   A) More in female
   B) Presentation is within three days
   C) Rectal biopsy is diagnostic
   D) Regular dilatation effective
14. Skip lesions with tuberculoid granuloma is seen in:
   A) Sarcoidosis
   B) Hodgkin's disease
   C) Ulcerative colitis
   D) Crohn's disease
15. Psudopolyps are features of:
   A) Crohn's disease
   B) Ulcerative colitis
   C) Coeliac disease
   D) Whipple's disease
16. Predisposing factors for gastric carcinoma include all/E
   A) Pernicious anaemia
   B) Blood group A
   C) Gastric polyp
   D) Hypercalcaemia
17. All are true for typhoid ulcer except
   A) Longitudinal
   B) Involve Peyer's patches
   C) Can perforate
   D) Heals with stricture formation
18. Premalignant conditions of oesophagus:
   A) Barret oesophagus
   B) Achalasia
   C) Post-ingestion of lye (alkaline burn)
   D) All of the above
19. Premalignant conditions of stomach
   A) Gastric polyp
   B) Hypertrophic gastritis
   C) Achlorhydria
   D) All of the above
20. Premalignant conditions of colon all/Except
   A) Ileocaecal tuberculosis
   B) Familial polyposis
   C) Villous adenoma
   D) Ulcerative colitis
21. Pseudomyxoma peritonei is seen with:
   A) Mucinous cysadenoma ovary
   B) Hepatoma
   C) Carcinoma appendix
   D) Carcinoma pancreas
22. Villous atrophy is a histological appearance, where small intestine has flat mucosa and crypt hypertrophy
   A) Coeliac disease
   B) Tropical sprue
   C) HIV enteropathy
   D) All of the above
23. Ormond's disease is:
   A) Intraabdominal desmoid
   B) Retroperitoneal fibrosis
   C) Retroperitoneal carcinomatosis
   D) Refractile mesenteritis.
24. Features of Crohn's disease are all except:
   A) Lymphoid hyperplasia
   B) Skip lesions
   C) Transmural involvement
   D) Crypt abscess
25. Most common site of carcinoma stomach
   A) Prepyloric
   B) Body of stomach
   C) Fundus
   D) Lesser curvature
26. Curling's ulcer is seen in:
   A) Burn patients
   B) Patients with head injury
   C) Zollinger Ellison syndrome
   D) Analgesic drugs

27. Which of the following is not related with carcinoma stomach?
   A) Blood group O
   B) Blood group A
   C) Smoked fish
   D) Nitrosamines
28. The presenting symptom of non-cirrhotic portal hypertension is:
   A) Chronic liver failure
   B) Ascitis
   C) Upper G I bleeding
   D) Encephalopathy
29. Jejunal biopsy is diagnostic in:
   A) Coeliac sprue
   B) Tropical sprue
   C) Whipple's disease
   D) Radiation enteritis
30. Paraneoplastic syndrome associated with oesophageal carcinoma is:
   A) Peripheral neuritis
   B) Sclerosing cholangitis
   C) Hypercalcaemia
   D) Cushing's syndrome

Answers

1. C) Plummer-Vinson syndrome: This condition commonly occurs in edentulous nourished middle-aged women with iron deficiency anaemia. Mucosa at the junction between oesophagus and hypopharynx may form "web like" projections into the lumen and lead to dysphagia.

2. D) Cigarette smoking is a major cause of oesophageal cancer in United States. The use of tobacco products including cigarettes, cigars, pipes, and chewing tobacco, is a major risk factor for oesophageal cancer. Someone who smokes at least a pack a day has twice the chance of getting adenocarcinoma of oesophagus than nonsmokers.

3. C) In cases of pernicious anaemia there is autoimmune atrophic gastritis. There is autoimmune destruction of gastric parietal cells leading to lack of intrinsic factor. The loss of gastric mucosal folds and thinning of the gastric mucosa recognize chronic atrophic gastritis grossly. In pernicious anaemia there are decreased number or absence of argentaffin cells, achlorhydria, and not associated with Helicobacter pylori infection.

4. B) There are two classes of antibodies seen in untreated celiac disease. Antibodies directed against a particular tissue in the body itself. The two main areas in the body which can be attacked by its own antibodies are the endomysial (the covering of muscle), and the reticulin (the framework for kidney and liver) Serology for anti-TGT (anti-tissue transglutaminase antibodies has superseded older serological test has a high sensitivity (99%) and specificity (> 90%) for identifying the celiac disease. Other tests include anti-endomysial antibody test, anti-gliadin and anti reticulin test.

5. D) Conditions associated with H. pylori are gastric carcinoma, MALTOMA and Barrett's oesophagitis.

6. B) Carcinoid tumours arise from neuroendocrine cells present in mucosa throughout gastrointestinal tract. The tumour arises from argentaffin cells.

Sites: Midgut and appendix 60 to 80%

Hind gut: Rectum 10 to 20%

Foregut: Oesophagus, stomach and duodenum 2-15%

7. D) Complications of duodenal ulcer include haemorrhage, perforation, scarring with obstruction. Incidence of malignant ulcer is very rare.

8. B) In a developing country like India, malignancy is the commonest cause of gastric outlet obstruction.

9. D) Pseudomyxoma peritonei is an uncommon tumour for its production of mucus in abdominal cavity. The disease is most commonly associated with cancer of the appendix.

10. D) Dysphagia is the medical term for the symptom of difficulty in swallowing. Causes of dysphagia include:

1. Neurological causes: Parkinson's disease, multiple sclerosis, progressive bulbar palsy
2. Muscular: Myaesthenia gravis, muscular dystrophy, achlasia
3. Carcinoma oesophagus
4. Extrinsic compression of oesophagus
5. Plummer-Vinson syndrome (syndrome in iron deficiency anaemia)

11. B) The commonest site of carcinoma oesophagus is:

1. Middle third of oesophagus
2. Near the level of diaphragm (Lower third)
3. Upper third at about the level of cricoid cartilage
4. Post cricoid cartilage.

12. A) In chronic gastric ulcer in the lesser curvature, a saddle shaped ulcer is often formed and after healing it may result in hour-glass contraction of the stomach.

13. C) Males are commonly affected. Male female ratio is 4:1. Male patients also have a shorter aganglionic segment than female patients.

14. D) Skip lesions are seen in Crohn's disease. Other features include:

1. The inflammatory process typically involves all layers of the gut wall (i.e. it is transmural) and may extend into the mesentery.
2. The mucosa shows diffuse hyperemia, acute inflammation, abnormal villus pattern and shallow aphthous ulceration.
3. Ill -defined clumps of lymphocytes and plasma cells are scattered in the submucosa and subserosa. Germinal center is present in the exudate.
4. Discrete, noncaseating granulomas, mostly in the submucosa, is also often present. In many cases ulceration is associated with metaplasia of gastric type.
5. The regional lymph nodes show noncaseating granulomas or reactive hyperplasia with prominent lymphoid follicles.

15. B) In ulcerative colitis the repeated cycle of ulceration, alternating with the deposition of granulation tissue during the healing phase, results in the development of raised areas of inflamed tissue that resemble polyps. However, these lesions are not neoplastic i.e., (true polyps), but inflammatory tissue and are called pseudopolyps.

16. D) Aetiology and predisposing factors

Gastric carcinoma is rare in tropical Africa, but extremely common in Japan, Chile, and some parts of Asia, Finland and Iceland. In India, it is common in Andhra pradesh, Chennai, and Assam.

1. **Age**: Carcinoma of stomach occurs between the ages of 40 t0 60 years. The average age is 38 years.
2. **Sex**: There is preponderance in males, M: F ratio is 2:1 in high-risk areas.
3. **Diet**: High intake of starch may alter the pattern of gastric secretion and predispose to cancer of stomach. Smoked and salted meats, rice dusted with asbestos containing talc, low green vegetables predisposes to carcinoma stomach. Tobacco smoke, tobacco juice and consumption of alcohol have carcinogenic effect on gastric cancer. Nitrates in food preservative get converted to carcinogenic nitrites and nitroso compounds by the action of bacteria. Widespread use of refrigeration may contribute in declining incidence. Intake of vitamin C, vitamin E and beta carotene protects against the ill affects of nitrites.

4. The frequency of gastric carcinoma is greater in adults suffering from pernicious anaemia.
5. **H. Pylori**: Chronic gastritis associated with H. pylori infection remains a major risk factor for gastric atrophy, intestinal metaplasia, and ultimately dysplasia and cancer.
6. **Genetic**: There may also be a genetic predisposition, for there is a slightly increased risk in people of blood group A. Carcinoma of stomach occurring simultaneously in identical twins has been reported. HNPCC genes involved in DNA repair systems when mutated can lead to a higher incidence of gastric carcinoma. C ras is rarely mutated, but common mutations include C met, K sam and erb.
7. **Premalignant**: The incidence is increased by about 10 times in individuals with atrophic gastritis. Precancerous lesions in stomach include hypochlorhydria, intestinal metaplasia, biliary reflux after partial gastrectomy, adenomatous polyps, Menetrie's disease and Barrett's esophagus.

17. D) There is no stricture formation in typhoid ulcer of small intestine.

Macroscopically: An ulcer involving a whole Peyer's patch is typically oval and placed with its long axis in that of the bowel. Its margins are thin, soft, ragged and undermined, while its floor, if completed cleaned of debris is fairly smooth and may show the transverse markings of the inner muscular coat.

Complications

1. Perforation: Perforation of the typhoid ulcer is seen in only 2% of cases. Perforation of the last 3 to 4 feet of the terminal ileum is seen usually in the third week of illness. The site of perforation is longitudinally placed ulcers at the sites of Peyer's patches. Peritonitis develops and the treatment is by closure of perforation.
2. Haemorrhage: Typhoid causes ulceration of the mucosa of the ileum. Bleeding can be small and intermittent or massive. Characteristically, the patient passes maroon coloured stools. Acquired thrombocytopaenia and deficiency of hepatically derived clotting factors secondary to typhoid hepatitis may cause further bleeding.
3. Paralytic ileus is probably the commonest complication of typhoid and is associated with distention of abdomen.
4. Cholecystitis occurs and can be severe enough to cause perforation of gall bladder. Gallstone may contain typhoid bacilli and a carrier state can develop in some patients.
5. Osteomyelitis
6. Typhoid spine
7. Cystitis, pyelitis, and epididymo-orchitis.
8. Typhoid lobar pneumonia is a rare complication occurring in the second and third week of illness.

18. D) Lye is a caustic, alkaline chemical that is useful for many purposes but also is hazardous. It can dissolve sticky substances such as fat and has high degree of reactivity with other materials. Modern lye typically is the chemical sodium hydroxide.

Premalignant conditions of oesophagus are:

1. Chronic alcoholism
2. Tobacco smoking
3. Food containing nitrosamines
4. Plummer-Vinson syndrome
5. Ingestion, of usually suicidal, of corrosive chemical such as lye or other alkalis and acids
6. Barret oesophagus

7. **Achalasia oesophagus**: The most serious aspect of achalasia is the hazard of development of carcinoma of the oesophagus, said to occur in 2 to 7% of these o-patients.

19. D) Premalignant conditions of stomach include:
- Autoimmune gastritis
- Chronic gastric ulcer
- H. pylori, especially if treated with PPI without irradication of H. pylori
- Gastric polyp
- Hypertrophic gastritis
- Atrophic gastritis
- Achlohydria or hypochlorhydria
- Intestinal metaplasia
- Post-gastrectomy
- Post-vagotomy
- Post-gastrojejunostomy

20. A) Tuberculosis is not a precancerous condition

Premalignant conditions of colon include:
- Hereditary cancer syndrome: FAP, Gardner's, HNPCC (hereditary nonpolyposis colorectal cancer)
- Chronic inflammatory bowel disease, especially chronic extensive ulcerative colitis
- Sporadic adenomatous polyps, especially villous and tubulovillous polyps.

21. A) Pseudomyxoma peritonei is a rare malignant growth characterized by progressive accumulation of mucus secreting (mucinous) tumour cells within the abdomen and pelvis.

Majority of these cells are associated with appendiceal carcinomas, appendix adenoma, appendiceal cyst. Other primary sites that have been reported including colon, rectum, stomach, gallbladder, bile ducts, small intestine, urinary bladder, lung, breast, fallopian tube and pancreas.

Causes of pseudomyxoma peritonei:
- Malignant appendiceal tumour
- Appendix adenoma
- Malignant large bowel tumour
- Malignant large bowel cyst
- Adenocarcinoma (mucus secreting)
- Malignant large bowel peritoneal carcinomatosis
- Mucinous cystadenoma
- Mucinous cystadenocarcinoma
- Colloid carcinoma
- Pseudomyxoma ovarii
- Disseminated peritoneal adenomucinosis
- Peritoneal mucinous carcinoma
- Peritoneal carcinomatosis

22. D) Villous atrophy is a histological appearance, where small intestine has flat mucosa and crypt hypertrophy.

Causes of villous atrophy
- Coeliac disease
- Post-enteritis syndrome
- Cow milk protein intolerance
- Giardiasis
- Immune deficiency states
- Eosinophilic gastroenteritis
- HIV enteropathy
- Tropical sprue
- Soya allergy

23. B. Retropertoneal fibrosis or Ormond's disease is a feature in the proliferation of fibrous tissue in the retroperitoneum, the compartment of the body containing the kidneys, aorta, renal tract and various other structures.

Their associations with various immune related conditions and response to immunosuppression have led to speculations as the autoimmune etiology of idiopathic PRF.

One third of cases are secondary to malignancy, medication (beta-blockers), aortic aneurysm or certain infections, Riedel's thyroiditis, previous radiotherapy and sarcoidosis.

24. D) Crypt abscesses are seen in ulcerative colitis.

Crohn's disease: The disease characteristically shows **skip-lesions,** affecting a segment of the small bowel with areas of normal mucosa in between. The affected mucosa usually shows linear or laciform ulceration with intervening mucosal swelling producing a cobblestone appearance. The lumen is narrowed. Often fat from the mesentery beneath the serosa surround the involved segment of bowel the lesion feels like a hosepipe or a dead eel.

Microscopically:

1. The inflammatory process typically involves all layers of the gut wall (i.e. it is **transmural**) and may extend into the mesentery.
2. The mucosa shows diffuse hyperemia, acute inflammation, abnormal villus pattern and shallow aphthous ulceration.
3. Ill -defined clumps of lymphocytes and plasma cells are scattered in the submucosa and subserosa. Germinal center is present in the exudate.
4. Discrete, noncaseating granulomas, mostly in the submucosa, is also often present. In many cases ulceration is associated with metaplasia of gastric type.
5. The regional lymph nodes show noncaseating granulomas or reactive hyperplasia with prominent lymphoid follicles.

25. A) Most common site of carcinoma stomach is prepyeloric region.

26. A) Curling's ulcers are seen in the posterior aspects of the first part duodenum in severe burn. When reduced plasma volumes leads to sloughing of the gastric mucosa.

27. A) It has been observed that persons belonging to O group are liable to peptic ulcers. Nitrates in food preservative get converted to carcinogenic nitrites and nitroso compounds by the action of bacteria.

There may also be a genetic predisposition. There is a slightly increased risk in people of blood group A.

Smoked and salted meats and fish, rice dusted with asbestos containing talc, low green vegetables predisposes to carcinoma stomach.

28. C) Acute upper gastrointestinal bleed is the most common presenting symptom of extra-hepatic portal hypertension.

Esophagio-gastric varices are present in 85 to 95% of cases. 70% of patients are with variceal bleeding.

29. B) Jejunal mucosa in tropical sprue with altered mucosal pattern due to joining of villi to form leaves and short ridges. Altered mucosal patterns were prevalent and more marked in jejunum than ileum. Other features of edema, crowding villi and reduction in height of villi is also seen frequently.

30. C) Paraneoplastic syndrome associated with oesophageal carcinoma is hypercalcaemia.

Peripheral neuropathy is seen in patients with lung carcinoma

Small cell carcinoma of lung is associated with Cushing's syndrome.

chapter 10

ENDOCRINE PATHOLOGY

1. Oncocytes are seen in
   A) Pituitary
   B) Thyroid
   C) Pancreas
   D) Thymus
2. Zollinger-Ellison syndrome is due to tumour of which cell?
   A) G cells
   B) Alpha cells
   C) Beta cells
   D) PP cells
3. In medullary carcinoma of thyroid marker is?
   A) Calcitonin
   B) TSH
   C) T_3 T_4 TSH
   D) Alphafetoprotein
4. Most common islet cell tumour in MEN 1 is:
   A) Gastrinoma
   B) Beta cells
   C) Glucagonoma
   D) Somatostatinoma
5. Medullary carcinoma of thyroid arises from?
   A) Cells lining the acini
   B) Capsule of thyroid
   C) Parafollicular cells
   D) Stroma of the glands
6. The most common histologic type of thyroid tumour is:
   A) Follicular carcinoma
   B) Papillary carcinoma
   C) Medullary carcinoma
   D) Anaplastic carcinoma
7. Conn's syndrome is:
   A) Adrenal hyperplasia
   B) Adrenal carcinoma
   C) Adrenal adenoma
   D) All of the above
8. Commonest cause of hyperparathyroidism is:
   A) Parathyroid adenoma
   B) Parathyroid carcinoma
   C) Chronic renal failure
   D) Parathyroid hyperplasia
9. Waterhouse-Friderichsen syndrome is characterized by except:
   A) High blood pressure
   B) DIC
   C) Purpura
   D) Haemorrhagic adrenalitis
10. Stomatostatin is secreted by:
    A) Alpha cells
    B) Insulinoma
    C) Delta cells
    D) D1 cells
11. Pheochromocytoma predominantly secretes?
    A) Norepinephrine
    B) Epinephrine
    C) Dopamine
    D) DOPA

12. Hurthle cells are seen in?
    A) Hashimoto's thyroiditis
    B) Follicular cell carcinoma
    C) Hurthle cell adenoma
    D) All of the above
13. Cushing's disease presents with
    A) Increased ACTH, increased cortisol
    B) Decreased ACTH, decreased cortisol
    C) Increased ACTH, decreased cortisol
    D) Increased catecholamines
14. Following statements about glucagon is true except:
    A) It is positive isotope
    B) It is produced by β cells of pancreas
    C) Stimulates the production of free fatty acids in the blood
    D) Its release is increased in salivation
15. Deficiency of 17-hydroxylase in the adrenal glands leads to a decreased level of hormone:
    A) Testosterone
    B) Thyroxine
    C) Cortisol
    D) Estrogen
16. Screening method for medullary carcinoma thyroid is?
    A) Serum calcitonin
    B) Serum calcium
    C) Serum ALP
    D) Serum acid phosphatase
17. Most common malignant tumour of infancy is:
    A) Malignant lymphoma
    B) Neuroblastoma
    C) Wilm's tumour
    D) Hepatoblastoma
18. Cushing's triad includes all except:
    A) Hypertension
    B) Bradycardin
    C) Hypothermia
    D) Irregular respiration
19. Zollinger Ellison syndrome is:
    A) Beta cell tumour
    B) Non-beta cell tumour
    C) Carcinoma
    D) Glucagonoma
20. Following is the feature of Addison's disease:
    A) Hypoglycaemia
    B) Hypokalemia
    C) Increased catabolism of protein
    D) Hypernitremia
21. A patient with centripetal obesity, acne, and hirsuitism. Most likely diagnosis is:
    A) Cushing's syndrome
    B) Diabetes mellitus
    C) Hypogonadism
    D) Hypothyroidism
22. The ratio of T3 : T4 secreted by thyroid gland is:
    A) 1: 5
    B) 1:20
    C) 1: 8
    D) 1:10
23. Commonest cause of abdominal mass in neonate is:
    A) Neuroblastoma
    B) Wilm's tumour
    C) Leukaemia
    D) Non-Hodgkin's lymphoma
24. Parafollicular cell related to:
    A) Thyroid gland
    B) Parathyroid gland
    C) Pituitary gland
    D) Pineal gland
25. Following signs and symptoms are associated with somatostatoma except:
    A) Diabetes mellitus
    B) Diarrhoea and steatorrhoea
    C) Migratory necrolytic erythema
    D) Gallstone
26. Psammoma bodies may be seen in the following except:
    A) Follicular carcinoma thyroid
    B) Meningioma
    C) Papillary carcinoma thyroid
    D) Serous cystadenoma thyroid

27. The causes of hypothyroidism include the following except:
    A) Hashimoto's thyroiditis
    B) Cretinism
    C) Irradiation
    D) Diffuse Subacute lymphocytic thyroiditis
28. Crooke's hyaline change is observed in the cells of:
    A) Adrenal cortex
    B) Acidophils of anterior pituitary
    C) Basophils of anterior pituitary
    D) Adrenal medulla
29. Zebra bodies are present in the pituitary in which of the following diseases?
    A) Cushing's syndrome
    B) Hand-Schuller-Christian disease
    C) Hurler's syndrome
    D) Simmond's syndrome
30. Commonest cause of Addison's disease is:
    A) Amyloidosis
    B) Histoplasmosis
    C) Autoimmune adrenalitis
    D) Tuberculosis
31. Which of the following does not usually show an association with pheochromocytoma?
    A) Cerebellar angioblastoma
    B) Conn's disease
    C) Medullary carcinoma thyroid
    D) Hyperparathyroidism
32. Pheochromocytoma occurs in the following locations except:
    A) Adrenal medulla
    B) Adrenal cortex
    C) Bladder
    D) Thorax
33. Which of the following may not be associated with medullary carcinoma of thyroid?
    A) Neurofibromatosis
    B) Pheochromocytoma
    C) Marfan's syndrome
    D) Zollinger-Ellison syndrome
34. Risk factors of carcinoma pancreas are:
    A) Smoking
    B) Chronic pancreatitis
    C) Mutation of BRCA 2 gene
    D) All of the above
35. Pheochromocytoma is associated with:
    A) SturgeWeber syndrome
    B) von-Hippel-Landu
    C) Neurofibromatosis
    D) All of the above
36. HLA important in IDDM:
    A) HLA A3
    B) HLA-27
    C) HLA DRW3DR4
    D) HLA-B47
37. Salt and pepper appearance of skull is seen in:
    A) Hyperthyroidism
    B) Hypothyroidism
    C) Hyperparathyroidism
    D) Thalassaemia major
38. Balloning of sella is X-ray finding in:
    A) Hydrocephalus
    B) Empty sella syndrome
    C) Chromophobe adenoma
    D) Meningioma
39. Common cause of thyrotoxicosis is:
    A) Grave's disease
    B) Follicular adenoma
    C) Multinodular goiter
    D) Well-differentiated carcinoma
40. Osteitis fibrosa cystica is seen in:
    A) Hypoparathyroidism
    B) Hypothyroidism
    C) Hyperthyroidism
    D) Hyperparathyroidism
41. Amyloid in pancreas occurs in:
    A) Acute pancreatitis
    B) Chronic pancreatitis
    C) Type II diabetes mellitus
    D) Carcinoma pancreas

42. Most common cause of acute pancreatitis is:
   A) Biliary tract diseases
   B) Alcoholism
   C) Post-traumatic
   D) Idiopathic
43. Cushing's syndrome is due to hyperfunction:
   A) Thyroid gland
   B) Parathyroid gland
   C) Islet cell tumour
   D) Adrenal gland

Answers

1. B) Oncocytes are characterized as enlarged epithelial cells with abundant eosinophilic granular cytoplasm as a result of altered mitochondria. They are generally stain pink and are predominantly found in histological sections of thyroid gland affected with Hashimoto's thyroiditis.

2. A) Zollinger Ellison syndrome is caused by tumours, usually found in the head of the pancreas and the upper small bowel. These tumours produce the hormone gastrin and called gastrinomas. A non-beta islet cells cause Zollinger-Ellison syndrome, gastrin-secreting tumour of the pancreas. G cells are found deep within the gastric glands of the stomach antrum and occasionally in pancreas.

3. A) Medullary carcinoma thyroid is a form of thyroid carcinoma which originates from the parafollicular cells (C cells), which produce the hormone calcitonin. Serum calcitonin in patients with thyroid nodules can detect cases of unsuspected medullary carcinoma thyroid.

4. A) Gastrinomas are sporadic in approximately 70% of patients and are a part of the MEN-1 in 30%. Insulinoma well known islet cell tumour of pancreas. Approximately 10% are associated with MEN-1.

5. C) Medullary carcinoma of thyroid arises from parafollicular cells of thyroid.

6. B) Most common histiologic type of thyroid carcinoma is papillary carcinoma of thyroid. It constitutes more than 70% of thyroid cancer.

7. C) Primary hyperaldosteroidism has many causes, including adrenal hyperplasia, and adrenal carcinoma. When it occurs due to a solitary aldosterone-secreting adrenal adenoma it is known as Conn's syndrome.

8. A) A parathyroid adenoma is a non-cancerous (benign) tumour of parathyroid gland. The most common cause of parathyroid adenoma is hyperparathyroidism.

9. A) Waterhouse-Friderichsen syndrome or haemorrhagic adrenalitis is a disease of adrenal glands most commonly caused by bacterium Neisseria meningitides. It is characterized by hypotension, disseminated rapid developing adrenocortical insufficiency.

10. C) Delta cells or D cells are somatostatin-producing cells. They can be found in the stomach, intestine, and the islets of Langerhans in the pancreas.

11. A) Pheochromocytoma is a rare catecholamine-secreting tumour derived from chromaffin cells. Most pheochromocytomas predominantly produce norepinephrine, unlike the normal adrenal medulla, which secrete epinephrine.

12. D) Hurthle cells are characterized as enlarged epithelial cells with abundant eosinophilic granular cytoplasm, as a result of altered mitochondria. They generally stain pink are predominantly found in histological sections are thyroid glands affected with Hashimoto's thyroiditis, follicular carcinoma, and Hurthle cell carcinoma.

13. A) Cushing's syndrome (also called hyperadrenocorticism is a hormone (endocrine) high levels of cortisol in the blood. Pituitary ACTH hypersecretion or (Cushing's syndrome) is a form of hyperpituitarism characterized by an abnormally high level of ACTH produced by anterior pituitary.

14. B) Glucagon is secreted and synthesized by alpha cells of the islet cells of pancreas.

15. A) 17-beta hydroxysteroid dehydrogenase deficiency is a condition that affects male sexual development. People with this condition are genetically male with X and Y chromosome in each cell, and they have male gonads (testes). Their bodies however do not produce enough of male sex hormone testosterone.

16. A) Medullary carcinoma is characterized by a high concentration of serum calcitonin. Routine measurement of serum calcitonin concentration has been advocated for detection of MCT among patients with nodular thyroid diseases.

17. B) Neuroblastoma is most common malignant tumour in infancy. 50% are under 2 years of age.

18. C) Cushing's triad is the triad of widening pulse pressure (rising systolic, declining diastolic), change in respiratory pattern (irregular respirations) and bradycardia.

19. B) Zollinger Ellison syndrome (ZES) is caused by a non-beta cell tumour, gastrin secreting tumour that stimulates the acid secreting cells of the stomach to maximal activity, with consequent gastrointestinal mucosal ulceration. The primary tumour is usually located in the duodenum, the pancreas, and abdominal lymph nodes but ectopic locations have been described (e.g., heart, ovary, gallbladder, liver and kidney).

20. A) Addison's crisis is characterized by sudden penetrating pain in legs, lower back or abdomen, severe vomiting, diarrhoea, resulting in dehydration, low blood pressure, hypoglycaemia, confusion, psychosis, slurred speech, severe lethargy, hypercalcaemia, convulsions, and fever.

21. A) Signs and symptoms of Cushing's syndrome are rapid weight gain, central obesity, moon face, hyperhidrosis, telangiectasia, red striae, hirsutism, baldness, hypercalcaemia, insomnia, libido, incompetence infertility, psychosis, anxiety and acne.

22. B) The thyroid hormone thyroxine (T4) and tridothyronine are tyrosine–based hormones produced by the thyroid gland primarily responsible for regulation of metabolism. The major form of thyroid hormone (T3:T4) in the blood is roughly is 1:20.

23. A) Neuroblastoma is the most common abdominal malignancy in infancy and the most common extracranial solid tumour of childhood. It is a poorly differentiated neoplasm derived from neural crest cells that typically affects infants and young children.

24. A) Para follicular cells (also called C cells) are cells of thyroid that produce and secrete calcitonin. They are located adjacent to the thyroid follicles and reside in the connective tissue. These cells are large and pale stain as compared with follicular cells or colloid.

25. C) Somatostatoma is a tumour of the delta cells of the endocrine pancreas that produce somatostatin. It is associated with diabetes mellitus, and abnormal glucose tolerance. It is a triad of diabetes mellitus, steatorrhoea, and gallstones, also associated with hyperchlorhydria. The tumour is commonly found in pancreas.

26. A) Psammoma bodies usually have a laminar, calcified, concentric appearance, are circular acellular and eosinophilic. They are thought to be remnants of degenerate papillary structure. Psammoma bodies are commonly seen in certain tumours such as papillary thyroid carcinoma, papillary renal cell carcinoma, serous papillary ovarian adenocarcinoma, endometrial carcinoma (papillary serous carcinoma), serous cystadenoma ovary (papillary type), meningioma, mesothelioma, and prolactinoma.

27. D) Subacute lymphocytic thyroiditis a previously unappreciated but surprising frequent problems can precipitate hyperthyroidism. The onset is within 3 to 6 months of delivery, and the condition is often mistaken for anxiety associated with the stress of caring for a new baby. Causes of hypothyroidism include, iodine deficiency, chronic autoimmune thyroiditis, thyroidectomy radiation, drugs (lithium), subacute thyroiditis, Hashimoto's thyroiditis.

28. C) Crook's hyaline change was studied by immunochemistry using an anti-adrenocorticotrophic hormone (ACTH) antiserum and five different antisera against cytokeratin. Crooke's hyaline appears in basophil cells of adenohypophysis in patients with hypercorticosolism, presumably as a part of negative feedback on corticotrophin secretion. Replacement of cytoplasmic granules of basophils cells of the anterior pituitary by homogenous hyaline material, a characteristic finding in Cushing's syndrome, but not present in the cells of a basophilic adenoma.

29. C) Hurler's syndrome, also known as mucopolysaccharidosis type I (MPS I). Hurler's disease is a genetic disorder that results in the buildup of mucopolysaccharides due to a deficiency of alpha-L iduronidase. Abnormal lysosomes are seen in the brain cell in mucopolysaccharide storage disorders known as Hurler's disease. The storage material accumulates in lysosomes appear striped hence the name "Zebra bodies".

30. C) Autoimmune adrenalitis is a form of adrenalitis, which is primarily caused by an autoimmune condition. It is commonest cause of Addison's disease. Other causes include tuberculosis of adrenal, cytotoxic destruction of adrenal, amyloidosis, fatty change, haemochromatosis, secondary tumours, thrombosis, embolism, and infection.

31. B) Multiple endocrine neoplasia, type 2A (MEN 2A) is a hereditary syndrome characterized by medullary carcinoma of thyroid, pheochromocytoma, hyperparathyroidism and occasionally cutaneous lichen planus. Several syndromes are associated with pheochromocytoma but Conn's syndrome has not been reported so far.

32. B) Pheochromocytoma arises from adrenal medulla. Other tumour arises from adrenal medulla is neuroblastoma. Extraadrenal pheochromocytomas are located in abdomen, thorax (10%) urinary bladder (1%) and carotid bifurcation. The tumours arises from adrenal cortex are adrenal adenoma and adrenal carcinoma.

The syndrome include, von-Recklinghausen's neurofibromatosis, von-Hippel-Landu disease, cerebellar angioblastoma, Albright syndrome, multiple mucocutaneous neuromas, and parathyroid adenomas.

33. D) Familial medullary carcinoma of the thyroid can be considered as part of a medullary thyroid carcinoma-pheochromocytoma syndrome. It is also associated with Marfan's syndrome and neurofibromatosis.

34. D) Risk factors of pancreatic carcinoma are smoking, hereditary chronic pancreatitis, and genetics. Smoking is one of the risk factors for developing pancreatic cancer. For heavy smokers, the risk of developing cancer 2 to 3 times more likely than a non-smoker.

Hereditary chronic pancreatitis is a rare genetic condition characterized by a long-term inflammation of the pancreas. The medical condition is associated with an increased risk of developing pancreatic cancer. People with a BARC 2 gene, responsible for developing breast cancer, have higher risk of pancreatic cancer.

35. D) Pheochromocytoma is associated with Sturge-Weber syndrome, VHL, neurofibromatosis, Sipple syndrome, cerebellar haemangioblastoma, renal cell carcinoma and tuberous sclerosis.

36. C) 60 to 70% of cases of insulin dependent diabetes mellitus are positive for HLA-DR3 or HLA-DR4.

HLA-B27 is associated with ankylosing spondylitis, post-gonococcal arthritis, and acute anterior uveitis.

Iron storage disease (haemochromatosis) has been tightly linked with HLA-3.

HLA- B47 is associated with 21-Hydroxylase deficiencies.

HLA-DR2 is associated with systemic lupus erythematosus, autoimmune hepatitis, primary Sjogren's syndrome

37. C) In cases of hyperparathyroidism radiographs distinctly show bone resorption and X-rays of the skull may depict an image often described as ground glass or salt and pepper skull.

Salt and pepper appearance of skull: Multiple small areas of resorption of skull in hyperparathyroidism results in mottled appearance like salt and pepper.

38. C) Plain roentgenographic changes typically include symmetrical ballooning of the sella, which still remains a closed configuration. Although the floor may be considerably thin, clinoids are usually not attenuated. In the anterioposterior view the sellar floor is symmetrical, in both position and bone thickness. Changes are characteristic of pituitary tumour including posterior displacement and deminéralization of the dorsum sellae and a double contour of the sellar floor; erosion of entire sella can also be seen.

39. A) Grave's disease

Etiology: The aetiology of Graves' disease is autoimmune, the exact mechanism that initiates the autoimmunity is not known.

PATHOLOGY

Macroscopically: Thyroid gland is smooth and soft, very vascular and has the appearance of muscle tissue.

Microscopically: The acini are irregular with marked hyperplasia of the epithelial cells. The epithelium is tall columnar in appearance. The reduction in the amount of colloid, and vacuoles are seen at the periphery of the acini (scalloping or moth eaten appearance). Infolding in the wall of the acini is a striking feature. Lymphocytes are present in the stroma and may form distinct follicles with germinal centers.

Clinical manifestations

Aetiology

Genetic: There is a well-defined association of HLA-DR3 and HLA-B89, so familial occurrences are known.

40. D) The skeletal manifestations of primary hyperparathyroidism may range from the relatively mild to crippling bone disease. There may be osteitis fibrosa cystica,

41. C) Amylin or islet amyloid polypeptide is a 37 residue peptide hormone secreted by â cells at the same time as insulin. Amyloid deposits deriving from islet amyloid polypeptide are commonly found in pancreatic islets cells suffering from diabetes mellitus type II or insulinoma. Amyloid appears as deposits of pink, amorphous material beginning in and around capillaries and between cells.

In advance stages, the islets may be virtually obliterated.

42. A) Most common cause of pancreatitis is:

Biliary tract calculi: Obstruction of the pancreatic duct may occur when a calculus becomes lodged in the ampulla of Vater.

Other causes

Alcoholism: Alcohol use is a major cause of acute pancreatitis. Most commonly, the disease develops in patients whose alcohol ingestion is habitual over 5 to 10 years. A direct toxic effect of alcohol in pancreatic acinar cells has been postulated.

Hypercalcaemia: as seen in hyperparathyroidism, among other conditions causes pancreatitis due to intraductal precipitation of calcium stones.

Hyperlipidemias on occasion can precipitate the onset of acute pancreatitis

Drugs: Probably associated with acute pancreatitis include chlorthiazide, hydrochlorthiazide, methadienova, metronidazole, nitrofurantoin, phenformin, and chemotherapeutic drugs.

Infections: Viral causes include mumps, Ebstein Barr, Cosackievirus, echovirus and measles. Bacteria causes include, mycobacterium tuberculosis, mycoplasma pneumoniae, salmonella, and campylobacteria.

Parasites: Round worms (Ascaris lumbricoides) which are normally resident in the upper jejunum, migrate towards the second part of duodenum, and enter the biliary passages or pancreatic duct, to give rise to a severe attack of pancreatitis. Many cases of roundworm pancreatitis have been reported from Kashmir.

Hereditary pancreatitis: This type of pancreatitis is an autosomal dominant gain-of- function disorder related to mutations of the cationic trypsinogen gene, which has an 80% penetrance. Mutations of this gene cause premature activation to trypsinogen to trypsin. In addition, the CFTR mutation plays a role in predisposing patients to acute pancreatitis a peculiar type of chronic pancreatitis occurs.

43. D) Cushing's syndrome is due to hyperfunction of adrenal glands. It is due to primary adrenocortical hyperplasia or neoplasia.

chapter 11

BREAST AND FEMALE GENITAL TRACT

1. Commonest presentation of choriocarcinoma is:
   A) Vaginal bleeding
   B) Abdominal pain
   C) Breathlessness
   D) Perforation of uterus
2. Ovarian tumour spreads primarily to which lymph nodes
   A) Para aortic lymph nodes
   B) Superficial inguinal lymph nodes
   C) Deep inguinal lymph nodes
   D) Node of Cloquet
3. Oestrogen replacement for postmenopausal symptoms cause an increase in?
   A) LDL
   B) Cholesterol
   C) VLDL
   D) Triglycerides
4. Pseudomyxoma peritonei is seen with
   A) Mucinous cystadenoma ovary
   B) Carcinoid appendix
   C) Endometrial carcinoma
   D) Ileal carcinoid
5. Herpes genitalis causes?
   A) Koilocytes in smear
   B) Atypical cells
   C) Carcinoma cervix
   D) Sterility
6. Commonest cause of post-menopausal bleeding is?
   A) Carcinoma endometrium
   B) Atrophic vaginitis
   C) Hyperplastic endometrium
   D) Endometrial polyp
7. Call-Exner bodies are characteristically seen in:
   A) Arrhenoblastoma
   B) Brenner tumour
   C) Dysgerminoma
   D) Granulosa cell tumour
8. Call-Exner bodies are a specific product of which of the following?
   A) Granulosa cells
   B) Theca cells
   C) Stromal cells
   D) All of the above
9. Which of the following conditions increase the risk of breast cancer?
   A) Apocrine metaplasia
   B) Calcium deposits
   C) Cysts
   D) Florid epithelial hyperplasia
10. Gynaecomastia may develop in:
    A) Cirrhosis of liver
    B) Klinefelter syndrome
    C) Digitalis therapy
    D) All of the above

11. Clue cells are seen in smear:
    A) Candidiasis
    B) Gardnerella vaginalis
    C) Herpes vaginalis
    D) Leptothrix
12. Investigation of a woman with a breast lump starts with:
    A) Fine needle aspiration cyto
    B) Mammography
    C) History and physical exam
    D) Excisional biopsy
13. Endometriosis choose correct answer:
    A) May occur as an implantation phenomenon after surgery
    B) Always cause dysmenorrhoea
    C) Does not cause under the age of eighteen
    D) Does not affect the ovaries
14. A single file infiltrating pattern of tumour cells in parallel arrays is classic for:
    A) Duct carcinoma in situ
    B) Infiltrating duct carcinoma
    C) Infiltrating lobular carcinoma
    D) Tubular carcinoma
15. Which of the following characteristics of breast carcinoma is associated with a better prognosis?
    A) Her2/neu protein overexpression
    B) Lymphovascular invasion
    C) High levels of hormone receptors
    D) Microscopic tumour of grade III
16. Cervicovaginal smear can diagnose except:
    A) Condyloma of the cervix
    B) Fungal infections
    C) Squamous cell carcinoma
    D) Ovarian carcinoid
17. Walthard rests are present in:
    A) Ovary
    B) Kidney
    C) Fallopian tube
    D) Uterus
18. Endometrial carcinoma
    Choose correct answer
    A) Lymph node spread does not occur
    B) Prevented by regular screening
    C) It is squamous type
    D) Is pre-invasive disease
19. Which of the following disorders may be mistaken for a carcinoma?
    A) Fibroadenoma
    B) Adenosis
    C) Gynaecomastia
    D) Fat necrosis
20. Which of the following breast lesions are noninvasive magnancies?
    A) Intraductal comedocarcinoma
    B) Tubular carcinoma
    C) Infiltrating duct carcinoma
    D) Medullary carcinoma
21. The most common cause of tubal damage is:
    A) Gonorrhoea
    B) Tuberculosis
    C) Chlamydia infection
    D) Bacterial vaginosis
22. Which one of the following endometrial lesion is thought to be associated with higher risk of developing endometrial carcinoma?
    A) Chronic endometritis
    B) Complex hyperplasia with atypia
    C) Complex hyperplasia without atypia
    D) Simple hyperplasia
23. Uterine myoma is least likely to undergo:
    A) Malignant change
    B) Hyaline change
    C) Calcification
    D) Red degeneration
24. Most common site of metastasis of choriocarcinoma is:
    A) Lung
    B) Vagina
    C) Liver
    D) Brain

25. Fibroid causes all of the following except:
A) Menstrual irregularities
B) Infertility
C) Abdominal mass
D) Amenorrhoea

26. Prenatal diagnosis of 16 weeks of pregnancy can be performed using all of the following except:
A) Amniotic fluid
B) Maternal blood
C) Chorionic villi
D) Fetal blood

27. Risk factors for the development of cervical cancers include all of the following except:
A) Smoking
B) Early onset of sexual activity
C) Multiple sexual partners
D) Unopposed oestrogen response

28. Common germ cell tumour of ovaries in post menopausal woman.
A) Brenner tumour
B) Dysgerminoma
C) Dermoid cyst
D) Mucinous cysadenoma

29. Type of malignancy in dermoid cyst of ovary is:
A) Transitional cell carcinoma
B) Adenocarcinoma
C) Squamous cell carcinoma
D) All of the above

30. DIC is common in:
A) Amniotic fluid embolism
B) Air embolism
C) Fat embolism
D) Thromboemboilsm

31. Peau'd orange in carcinoma breast is due to
A) Invasion of ligament Cooper
B) Sweat gland blockage
C) Lymphatic blockage
D) Lactiferous duct invasion

32. Virus involved in causing carcinóma cervix is:
A) Type 6
B) Type 2
C) Type 16
D) Type 21.

33. The percentage of leiomyoma which undergo malignant transformation:
A) 0.5%
B) 1.5%
C) 2%
D) 2.5%

34. Tumour marker in choriocarcinoma
A) CEA
B) HCG
C) α fetoprotein
D) β microglobulin

35. Which of the following is masculinizing tumour of ovary?
A) Granulosa cell tumour
B) Dysgerminoma
C) Dermoid cyst
D) Arrhenoblastoma

36. Commonest site of fibroid uterus is:
A) Submucus
B) Intramural
C) Subserous
D) Cervical

37. Endometrial hyperplasia is seen in:
A) Endodermal sinus tumour.
B) Dysgerminoma
C) Polycystic ovarian disease
D) Carcinoma cervix

38. Meigs' syndrome is commonly associated with:
A) Brenner tumour
B) Fibroma
C) Teratoma
D) Theca-cell tumour

39. Commonest vulval malignancy is:
A) Squamous cell carcinoma
B) Melanoma
C) Basal cell cacinoma
D) Adenocarcinoma

40. Solid ovarian tumours are all/Except
A) Dermoid

B) Struma ovarii
C) Serous cystadenoma
D) Granulosa cell tumour

41. Reinke crystals are seen in:
A) Papillary cystadenocarcinoma
B) Dermoid
C) Dysgerminoma
D) Hilus cell tumour

42. Bloody nipple discharge is usually associated with:
A) Breast abscess
B) Galactocele
C) Fibroadenoma breast
D) Intraduct papilloma

43. All of the following cause gynaecomastia except:
A) Klinefelter syndrome
B) Cirrhosis
C) Leprosy
D) Undescended testis

44. Cystosarcoma phylloids is:
A) Sarcoma breast
B) Giant fibroadenoma
C) Fibrocystic disease of breast
D) Adenosis breast

Answers

1. A) Commonest presentation of choriocarcinoma is irregular vaginal bleeding. If patient continues to bleed for longer than normal after a normal pregnancy or molar pregnancy, it may be symptom of this disease. Other symptoms include, abdominal swelling, anaemia, nausea and vomiting. In case of lung metastasis there is difficulty in breathing and sometimes chest pain. If it spreads to vagina then patient have excessive bleeding. Spread to brain causes headache, dizziness, and seizures. Uterine choriocarcinoma with spontaneous rupture have been reported.

2. A) Lymph node spread may occur early in the disease to para aortic lymph nodes.

3. D) Lipoproteins and oestrogen replacement therapy in post menopausal women: Abnormal lipid profile, per se, is an hypertriglyceridemia with oral oestrogen, all other parameters tend to be normalize following oestrogen replacement.

4. A) Pseudomyxoma peritonei is an uncommon tumour clinical syndrome characterized by the slow and progressive accumulation of peritoneal implants and mucinous ascitis. The disease is most commonly associated with cancer of the appendix and mucinous tumours of the ovary. Rupture of benign mucinous-adenoma leads to mucinous deposits on the peritoneum (pseudomyxoma peritonei). Symptoms may include abdominal or pelvic pain and/or bloating, distension, digestive disorders, weight changes, increased girth, and infertility.

5. B) Cytological smear in herpes genitalis shows presence of atypical cells. A definite epidemiological relationship between the viral infection and abnormal Papanicolaou smear and its frequent association with cytological changes in the cervix are noted. There is an evidence of premalignant changes or cytological smears suggesting atypical cervical cells.

6. B) Most common cause for post-menopausal bleeding is atrophic vaginitis, which is an inflammation of the lining of the vagina, caused by lower level of oestrogen. Other causes of post-menopausal bleeding are endometrial cancer, endometrial hyperplasia, endometrial and cervical polyps and oestrogen treatment.

7. D) Call-Exner bodies are characteristically seen in granulosa cell tumours. They are small spaces filled with eosinophilic fluid and basement membrane material between granulosa cells in maturing ovarian follicles and in ovarian tumour of granulosal origin. They may form a rosette like pattern.

8. A) Call-Exner bodies are a specific product of granulose cells, both normal and neoplastic. These consist of small, round masses of dense-pink inspissated material surrounded by rosette, of typical granulose cells.

9. D) Epithelial florid hyperplasia involves proliferation of epithelial layers usually three or more layers in thickness. Florid ductal hyperplasia pose only a slightly increase risk of breast cancer 1.5-2.0 times. Epithelial or ductal hyperplasia describes a proliferative condition that is manifested histologically as an increase in the cellularity of the epithelium of the terminal ducts. Epithelial hyperplasia ranges from mild though florid but typical. There is increase in epithelial layer lining, which distends the terminal ducts or ductules.

10. D) Gynaecomastia is the development of abnormally large mammary glands in males resulting in breast enlargement. Causes of gynaecomastia include Klinefelter syndrome, testicular atrophy, tumours, cirrhosis of liver, drugs, (digitalis, isoniconic acid hydrazine). It is a benign enlargement of the male breast resulting from a proliferation of glandular components.

11. B) Gardnerella vaginalis, a gram-negative rod, is a frequent cause of bacterial vaginitis. It manifests in smear as blue stained cocco-bacillary organism covering and imparting a grainy appearance of affected squamous cells (so called 'clue cells') against a clean background devoid of Doderlein bacilli.

12. C) Examination of breast lump starts with history and physical examination of patient. Painful and soft swelling suggests an abscess. Soft and movable lump shows benign swelling. Hard lump suggests sclerosing adenosis, fat necrosis and malignancy.

13. B) Endometriosis is a debilitating medical condition in females in which endometrial-like cells flourish in areas outside the uterine cavity, most commonly on the ovaries. The endometriosis has been found in abdominal incisional scars after surgery but it can be due to oestrogens, retrograde menstruation, mullaerianosis, coelomic metaplasia, genetics and transplantation, autoimmune diseases and birth defects. Endometriosis can occur at any age time after puberty. It is most commonly diagnosed in a women's twenties or early thirties, however, girls young as eight have been diagnosed with the disease. Dysmenorrhoea is a painful, sometimes disabling cramps, pain may get worse overtime (progressive pain) and also lower back pains linked to the pelvis.

14. C) The morphologic features of lobular carcinoma differ from those of ductal carcinoma. Infiltrating lobular carcinoma is characterized by small, rounded cells, that bland in appearance and have scant cytoplasm, which infiltrate the stroma in single file and surround benign tissues in a targeted manner. Infiltration typically does not destroy anatomic structures or incite a substantial connective tissue response.

15. C) Breast cancer cells may or may not have three important receptors: oestrogen receptor (ER), progesterone receptor (PR) and HER2/ neu. Cells with these receptors are called ER positive (ER+), ER negative (ER-), PR positive (PR+), PR negative (PR-), HER-2 positive (HER2+) and HER-2 negative. ER+ cancer cells depend on oestrogen for their growth, so they can be treated with drugs to reduce oestrogen e.g., tomoxifen and generally have a better prognosis. Generally HER-2+ have worst prognosis. Lymphovascular invasion and microscopic tumour of grade III have worst prognosis.

16. D) Cervicovaginal smears can diagnose condyloma (Human papilloma virus infection), herpes simplex infection, Gardnerella vaginalis infection, tuberculosis, filariasis, trichomonas, amoebiasis, candidiasis, aspergillosis and carcinoma. Carcinoid tumour of ovary can be diagnosed by fine needle aspiration cytology.

17. C) "Walthard cell rests", sometimes called Walthard cell nests are accumulation of the epithelial cells most commonly found in the peritoneum of the fallopian tubes, but also seen in the mesoovarian mesosalphinx-ovarian hilus.

18. B) Endometrial carcinoma metastasize to pelvic or para-aortic lymph nodes. It invades myometrium, cervical stromal invasion, adenexa, vagina, bladder and bowel. Early endometrial cancer is usually asymptomatic A routine Papanicolau test shows malignant cells in post-menopausal women. Endometrial carcinoma is adenocarcinoma.

19. D) Fat necrosis is a benign condition where fatty breast tissue swells and becomes tender, can occur spontaneously or as the result of injury to the breast. When the body attempts to repair damaged breast tissue, the affected area may sometimes be replaced with firm scar tissue. Fat necrosis may be mistaken as cancer clinically as well as on mammogram.

Fibroadenomas are solid, firm or rubbery benign lumps moves freely.

Gynaecomastia is an enlargement of male breast.

20. A) Tubular carcinoma, infiltrating duct carcinoma and medullary carcinoma are invasive malignancies of breast. Comedocarcinoma is a malignant intraductal neoplasm of the breast, in which the central cells degenerate and may be easily expressed from the cut surface of the tumour. Growth confined to the mammary ducts causes a better prognosis than do invasive breast lesions.

21. B) Pelvic tuberculosis is fairly common cause of tubal damage in India. The tuberculous bacteria reach the tubes from lung through blood stream and can cause irreparable tubal damage.

22. B) In general, any condition characterized by excessive oestrogenic stimulation is associated with some degree of endometrial hyperplasia associated with endometrial carcinoma. Endometrial hyperplasia is a histologic precursor of adenocarcinoma. The most severe changes are present in complex hyperplasia with atypia. Disorganization and crowding of glands, high mitotic activity, and nuclear atypia characterize this change. 25% of women with this form of hyperplasia develop adenocarcinoma.

23. A) Leiomyomas of uterus commonly undergo red degeneration, calcification and hyaline degeneration. Sarcomatous degeneration occurs in less than 1% of leiomyoma.

24. A) The most common site of systemic metastatic choriocarcinoma is lung. There may be coughing, bloody sputum, haemoptysis, and other symptoms. Lung.X-ray examination can be seen in sheets, cotton balls and nodular shadow. Other sites of metastatic choriocarcinoma are liver, brain, and vagina.

25. D) Symptoms that might be experienced by patients include: Heavy menstrual flows, bleeding between periods, pain, infertility, pelvic pressure, stress, urinary incontinence, and urethral obstruction.

26. D) Maternal serum testing is a non-invasive screen for trisomy-21, trisomy 18 and open neural tube defects. This is undertaken by measuring various fetal placental products in the serum at 15 to 20 weeks gestation. (Ideally 16 weeks). The standard genetic amniocentesis is undertaken after 16 weeks gestation and should always be done under continuous ultrasound guidance, Complications is much higher for early amniocentesis. Chorionic villus sampling or placental biopsy is undertaken either transabdominally or transcervically at 11-13 weeks gestation. Cordocentesis involves the insertion of needle into the umbilical cord for fetal blood sampling. Cordocentesis is performed at 18 weeks or after.

27. D) Prolonged periods of unopposed oestrogen are the main risk factor in carcinoma uterus. Women who smoke are about twice as likely as non-smokers to get cervical cancer.

28. C) The most common germ cell tumour is the benign cystic teratomas or dermoid cyst. Other germ cell tumours are malignant. They include dysgerminoma, yolk sac tumour and choriocarcinoma. The tumours usually observed in young women, are often bulky and composed of a variety of tissues derived from two or three embryonal layers, including skin, and its appendages which are often the dominant component. Dermoid cyst may occur in postmenopausal women.

29. C) Rarely dermoid cyst can be malignant and develop into squamous cell carcinoma.

30. A) Amniotic fluid embolism is a rare obstetric emergency in which it is postulated that amniotic fluid, fetal cell and hair and other debris enter the maternal circulation, causing cardio-respiratory collapse. DIC is a situation of inappropriate coagulation within blood vessels, which leads to the consumption of clotting factors thus resulting in the failure of clotting mechanism at the site of bleeding. Conditions precursors of DIC are retained placenta, amniotic fluid embolism, intrauterine with retained fetus and amniotic fluid embolism.

31. C) Peau'd orange describe the characteristic appearance of skin overlying a breast carcinoma. It is due to invasion of lymphatics by tumour producing obstruction and subsequently oedema of the underlying skin. This creates an orange peel appearance. Overlying a breast lump, this appearance is almost pathognomic of carcinoma.

32. C) Viruses like herpes simplex type –2 and Human papilloma virus type 16, 18, 31, 33, 35, 39, 45, 52, 56, 58, and 59 are more often associated indicating some causative role.

33. A) Malignant transformation (leiomyosarcoma) occurs in less than 0.5% of cases.

34. B) ONCOFOETAL ANTIGENS ASSOCIATED WITH MALIGNANCY

No.	Tumour antigen	Tumour
1.	Carcinoembryonic antigen CEA	Colorectal carcinoma, pancreatic carcinoma, gastric carcinoma, breast carcinoma, kidney tumours
2.	Alpha foetoprotein	Hepatocellular carcinoma, yolk sac tumour, embryonal carcinoma, polyembryoma, immature teratoma.
3.	Protein specific antigen	Carcinoma prostate
4.	Human chorio gonadotrophin	Trophoblastic tumours
5.	C A 125	Ovarian carcinoma, adenocarcinoma endometrium, pancreatic cancer, carcinoma colon, breast, lung.
6.	Tissue polypeptide antigen (TPA)	Cholangiocarcinoma
7.	CA 15-3, CA 549, CA 24-27	Breast carcinoma
8.	CA19-9, DU-PAN-2	Pancreatic carcinoma
9.	Beta-2 microglobulin	B-NHL, multiple myeloma, macroglobulinemia, CLL
10.	Nuclear matrix protein 22	Bladder carcinoma
11.	Squamous cell carcinoma antigen	Squamous cell carcinoma
12.	S100, HMB- 45	Melanoma

35. D) Arrhenoblastoma of the ovary is an ovarian tumour that releases the male hormone, testosterone or other hormones.

This is a rare tumour. It accounts for less than o.5% of all ovarian tumours.

The tumours are found in women of all age groups, but are most common in young women (ages 20 to 30 years).

The tumour releases male hormones, which causes the following symptoms in women.

- Deepening of the voice

- Increases acne
- Increased hair on the face and body
- Increased size of clitoris
- Male pattern baldness

36. B) **Sites**: Leiomyomas are present in myometrium of corpus uterine, lower uterine segment, uterine ligaments, and cervix.

Intramural: The leiomyomata are entirely within the myometrium and are most common type, unless they large they may be asymptomatic.

Subserosal: Tumour may project through the uterine serosa into the peritoneal cavity. Occasionally subserosal leiomyoma may become pedunculated and seen away from uterus described as wandering fibroid. Very rarely such a tumour becomes attached to the omentum or pelvic peritoneum loses its stalk to become a **parasitic leimyoma.**

Submucus: Occasionally tumours beneath the endometrium tend to bulge into the cavity and may eventually develop to form a fibroid polyp.

Cervical fibroids are located in the wall of cervix (neck of uterus).

37. C) Endometrial hyperplasia is a condition of excessive proliferation of the cells of the endometrium, or inner lining of the uterus. Most cases of endometrial hyperplasia result from high levels of oestrogens, combined with insufficient levels of the progesterone-like hormones, which ordinarily counteract oestrogens proliferating effects on this tissue.

This may occur in a number of setting including:

1. Obesity
2. Polycystic ovary syndrome
3. Granulosa cell tumour
4. Certain formulations of oestrogen replacement therapy

Endometrial hyperplasia is a significant risk for development or even co-existence of endometrial cancer.

38. B) Meig's syndrome also known as Meig's syndrome, is the triad of ascites, pleural effusion and benign ovarian tumour (fibroma). It resolves after the resection of the tumour. For reasons unknown, the pleural effusion is classically on right side.

39. A) Most important malignant tumour of the vulva is squamous cell carcinoma (85%). The remainders are adenocarcinoma (6%), melanoma (3%), and sarcoma (3%). It is rare and accounts for only 1-2 % of cancers of female genital tract.

About 75% of patients with squamous cell carcinoma of the vagina are over 50. Adenocarcinomas of the vagina more commonly affect younger women.

Women whose mothers took diethylstilbestrol (DES) during the first trimester of pregnancy are at increased risk for developing clear cell adenocarcinoma.

Verrucous carcinoma produces a warty, cauliflower-like growth that grows slowly; invading local tissues but almost never metastasizes.

Sarcoma botryoids of the vagina is a rare type of cancer that mainly occurs in infancy and childhood.

40. C) Causes of solid ovarian tumours

I. Benign tumours
1. Fibroma
2. Adenofibroma
3. Brenner's tumour

II. Malignant tumours
1. Carcinoma- adenoid carcinoma
2. Krukenberg's tumour

III. Tumours with endocrine dysfunction
1. Granulosa cell tumour
2. Thecoma (theca cell tumour)
3. Arrhenoblastoma
4. Dysgerminoma
5. Gynandroblastoma

41. D) Reinke Crystals: In Leydig cells lipofuscin pigment and rod shaped crystal like structures 3 to 20 micrometres in diameter (Reinke crystals) are found. Reinke crystals are seen in hilus cell tumour of the ovary

42. D) **Intraduct papilloma**: It is found near the age of menopause but occasionally in younger women. A discrete benign papillary tumour arises in a mammary duct. Woman presents with bleeding per nipple.

Macroscopically: They vary in size from 5 cm or more in diameter. When large, they may partially or totally occlude the duct in which they are located and produce a palpable clinical mass. Multiple papillomas (duct papillomatosis) represent a rather widespread hyperplasia and may be premalignant.

Microscopically: The tumour is typically characterized by orderly, often glandular growth pattern, well developed fibrovascular stalks minimal cellular pleomorphism; little hyperchromasia; low mitotic activity; foci of apocrine metaplasia, necrosis and lack of cribriform pattern. It is a precancerous condition and malignant changes may occur forming duct carcinoma.

43. C) Gynaecomastia is the development of abnormally large mammary glands in males resulting in breast enlargement. Causes of gynaecomastia include Klinefelter syndrome, testicular atrophy, tumours, cirrhosis of liver, drugs, (digitalis, isoniconic acid hydrazine). It is a benign enlargement of the male breast resulting from a proliferation of glandular components.

44. B) Cystosarcoma phylloides are variants of fibroadenoma, developing from fibroadenoma of usual type in elderly women and may attain a huge size. They are well circumscribed, lobulated and often cystic. They often distend the skin and form a fungating mass by ulceration of the skin.

chapter 12

MALE GENITAL SYSTEM

1. Seminoma corresponds to mass in ovary is:
   A) Granulosa cell tumour
   B) Dysgerminoma
   C) Thecoma
   D) Endodermal sinus tumour
2. Klinefelter syndrome is characterised:
   A) Gynaecomastia
   B) Azoospermia
   C) Increased urinary gonadotrophins
   D) All of the above
3. Acute orchitis is usually not caused by:
   A) Mumps
   B) Small pox
   C) Tuberculosis
   D) Scarlet fever
4. The important diagnostic microscopic feature in carcinoma of prostate is:
   A) Increased mitosis
   B) Proliferation of glandular epithelium
   C) Invasion of perineural lymphatics
   D) Back-to-back arrangement of the glands
5. Reinke crystalloids are seen in:
   A) Adenomatoid tumour
   B) Leydig cell tumour
   C) Polyembryoma
   D) Teratoma
6. Recent studies provide evidence that a hereditary prostate cancer susceptibility gene is likely to be contained in chromosome:
   A) 1 q
   B) 8p
   C) 10q
   D) 16q
7. The most common paratesticular mass is:
   A) Hydrocele
   B) Adenomatoid tumour
   C) Leiomyosarcoma
   D) Rhabdomyosarcoma
8. Which is the most type of tumour found in children?
   A) Seminoma
   B) Lymphoma
   C) Yolk sac tumour
   D) Teratocarcinoma
9. Germ cell tumour common in men over the age of 50:
   A) Choriocarcinoma
   B) Teratomas
   C) Endodermal sinus tumour
   D) Spermatocytic seminoma
10. Yolk sac tumour typically secretes:
    A) AFP
    B) B-HCG
    C) PLAP
    D) LDH
11. PSA is increased in:
    A) Benign prostatic hyperplasia
    B) Prostatitis
    C) Carcinoma prostate
    D) All of the above

12. Features of Sertoli cell only syndromes are except:
A) Infertility
B) Azoospermia
C) Gynaecomastia
D) Testicular atrophy
13. Leydig cell hyperplasia occurs in following conditions except:
A) Klinefelter syndrome
B) Cryptorchidism
C) Male pseudohermaphroditism
D) Congenital adrenal hyperplasia
14. Schiller-Duval body is seen in:
A) Seminoma
B) Yolk sac tumour
C) Teratoma
D) Lymphoma
15. Tumour having same histological features are seen in:
A) Ovary
B) Pineal and suprasellar location
C) Mediastinum
D) All of the above
16. Absence of fructose in semen indicates
A) Obstruction of vas
B) Obstruction of ejaculatory duct
C) Testicular failure
D) Prostate atrophy
17. Microscopic changes in atrophic testis includes all except:
A) Thickening of basement membrane of tubules
B) Absence of germ cells in tubules
C) Decrease number of Leydig cells
D) No change in Sertoli cells.
18. Features of carcinoma penis are all except:
A) Circumcision soon after birth provides immunity
B) Metastasize to inguinal lymph nodes
C) Surgery is treatment of choice
D) Transitional cell carcinoma
19. Ectopic testis is found in all locations except:
A) Lumbar
B) Perineal
C) Intraabdominal
D) Inguinal

Answers

1. B) Seminoma (pure seminoma) is a germ cell tumour of testis originates from the germinal epithelium of the seminiferous tubules. Primitive, unipotential germ cells are the precursors to ovarian dysgerminomas and their testicular analog, the seminoma.

2. D) Klinefelter syndrome is characterized by hypogonadism, gynaecomastia, azoospermia, testicular atrophy and increased gonadotrophic production. The basic karyotype is 46 XXY

3. C) Tuberculosis is a chronic inflammation not an acute infection. Acute orchitis may be a complication of systemic infections like mumps, smallpox, scarlet fever, diphtheria, dengue fever, typhus, and pneumonia.

4. C) Well differentiated adenocarcinoma of the prostate, may be histiologically difficult to distinguish from nodular hyperplasia. In these cases, the important diagnostic feature is the invasion of perineural spaces, capsular infiltration and vascular emboli.

5. B) Reinke crystalloids are rod shaped crystalline structures with pointed or rounded ends present in the interstitial cells of the testis (Leydig cells) and ovary. Crystalloids of Reinke are pathognomic of Leydig cell tumour.

6. A) Hereditary prostate cancers is a genetic form of prostate cancer. There are two known patterns of simple Mandelian inheritance in prostate cancer. These patterns are autosomal dominant and X-linked. A gene linked to an autosomal dominant and form of prostate cancer was mapped to the long q arm of chromosome 1. The gene is called HPC gene (hereditary prostate cancer-1). It has been located on the long arm of chromosome 1q24-25. Another gene responsible for hereditary prostate cancer has also been found on chromosome in region Xq27-28. The gene is called HPC X (hereditary prostate gene on the X).

7. B) Adenomatoid tumour is the most common tumour of the epididymis and spermatic cord. It may be asymptomatic or present as a painless scrotal mass in the region of the head of the epididymis. The cut surface of tumour is firm, white-grey, and homogenous. Paratesticular mass include spermatic granuloma, hydrocele and spermatocele. Other benign lesions are lipomas, adenomatoid tumours, leiomyomas, lymphoma, lymphangiomas, cystadenomas of the epididymis fibrous pseudotumours, neurofibromas, and myxomas. Malignant tumours included are rhabdomyosarcomas, fibrosarcoma, liposarcoma, angiosarcoma, malignant fibrosarcoma, leiomyosarcomas, mesotheliomas, and myxoid chondrosarcomas.

8. C) Seminoma, lymphoma and teratocarcinoma occur in fourth and fifth decades. Yolk sac tumour is most common tumour in children.

Other names are endodermal sinus tumours, infantile embryonal carcinoma, or orchioblastoma.

Yolk sac tumour resembles the yolk sac of the developing embryo.

Macroscopically: On cut section, the lesions tend to be yellow-grey, focally cystic, and solid masses of variable consistency.

Microscopically: A tumour characterized by cells of primitive appearance, growing typically in a loose vacuolated network. Reticular, tubular papillary, and solid patterns may be present. The tumour cells assume a delicate reticular (lace like) pattern or a papillary pattern in which structures that resemble glomeruli (glomeruloid or Schiller Duval bodies) are present. Many of cells contain and secrete small hyaline globules of alpha-fetoprotein.

9. D) Spermatocytic seminoma is a rare tumour, comprising only 1 to 2% of all testicular germ cell tumours. Men presenting with this tumour are generally 50 to 60 years old. Testicular teratomas occur in children and adults. Choriocarcinoma occurs most commonly in men aged 20-30 years.

10. A) Endodermal sinus tumour, also known as yolk sac tumour, is a member of the germ cell tumour group of cancers. It is more common in children under 3 years. These cells secrete alpha-fetoprotein, which can be detected in tumour tissue, serum, CSF, and urine.

11. D) Prostate specific antigen is a protein found in prostate cells. It can be detected in at a low level in the blood of all adult men. The normal value for total PSA is considered to be less than 4.0ng/ml

The test is done to screen prostate cancer. Several conditions besides cancer can cause the PSA level to rise including benign prostatic hyperplasia, prostatitis, recent catheterization or cystoscopy, and urinary tract infection.

12. C) Sertoli cell only syndrome, also called germ cell aplasia, describes a condition of the testis in which only Sertoli cells line the seminiferous tubules. The characteristics of Sertoli cell only syndrome are:

1. Semen analysis demonstrates azoospermia,
2. The testis may present with marked atrophy.
3. Patients with Sertoli cell only syndrome exhibit normal virilization without gynaecomastia.
4. Typically men with Sertoli cell only syndrome present between ages 20-40 years for evaluation of infertility.

13. C) Histologically Leydig cell hyperplasia is characterized by an increased number of testicular Leydig's cells with increased nucleoli, decreased lipofuscin, and decreased smooth endoplasmic reticulum. Causes of Leydig cell hyperplasia include cryptorchidism, congenital adrenal hyperplasia, hCG production by germ cell tumours or choriocarcinoma, pituitary abnormalities, Klinefelter syndrome, exogenous hCG therapy, and antiandrogen therapy for prostate cancer. There is Leydig cell hypoplasia in male hermaphroditism.

14. B) A Schiller-Duval body is a cellular structure seen by microscope in yolk sac tumours (endodermal sinus tumour) which are most common testicular tumours and if found are pathognomic. Schiller-Duval bodies are said to resemble glomerulus.

15. D) Other sites of histologically similar tumours as seminoma are ovary (dysgerminoma), pineal and suprasellar location and mediastinum.

16. B) Fructose in semen emanates mainly from the seminal vesicles, with a minor contribution from the corresponding secretory epithelium in the ampullatory part of the vas deferens. The secretion is androgen dependent. Fructose in semen is used as marker for the secretory contribution of the seminal vesicles to ejaculate or to characterize the origin of slit ejaculate fractions.

The content of 13.9 μmol fructose or more preejaculate indicates normal secretory contribution from the seminal vesicles to the ejaculate.

A content less than 13.0 μmol indicated a low androgen-specific contribution of vesicular fluid to ejaculate. This can be seen after a short time of abstinence, in partially hypogonadal men, and in men where emission or ejaculation is impaired. Emission can be hindered by neuromuscular diseases, post-surgery and by drugs and also due to obstruction in the ejaculatory ducts or temporarily by an inflammation in the vesicles or in the prostate.

17. C) Leydig cells are increased in number. Seminiferous tubules contain sertoli cells, but none of characteristics cells of spermatogenesis are seen. The basement membrane appears thicker than normal.

18. D) **It is a squamous cell carcinoma** presenting as an ulcerative, proliferative or an infiltrative lesion over the glans, coronal sulcus, frenum or the inner aspect of the prepuce.

Very rarely adenocarcinoma arising in glands of corona and frenum may occur.

Squamous cell carcinoma of penis represents about 1% of cancers in males in USA. Incidence is extremely rare among Jews and Moslems.

It is more common in India due to poor personal hygiene. **Circumcision done in infancy seems to prevent the occurrence of this carcinoma.** Smegma is considered to have carcinogenic effect. Predisposing causes of carcinoma penis includes phimosis, chronic balanitis and HPV infection. Premalignant lesions of penis are Bowen's disease, erythroplasia of Queyrat's and Bowenoid papulosis.

Two forms of growth occur;

1. Ulcer with sloughing base and hard rolled edges, usually it is adherent to underlying tissues.
2. Soft cauliflower growth.

Modes of spread of carcinoma penis

1. Local spread: Spread locally by infiltrating erectile tissue. Involvement of urethra is less common
2. **Lymphatic spread to inguinal lymph nodes,** and later retroperitoneal nodes.
3. Haematogenous metastases are uncommon and occur very late.

Penile intraepithelial neoplasia (PIN): It may develop as non-invasive carcinoma in situ form (Queyrat's erythroplasia), presenting as a red plaque. Many cases are associated with human papilloma virus infection.

Surgery is treatment of choice.

19. C) Common locations of ectopic testis are:

1. Perineal
2. Femoral canal
3. In the superficial inguinal pouch which lies anterior to the external oblique appearance at root of the penis.
4. Pubis
5. Contralateral scrotal pouch. Hence the testicle may be found in regions not in the usual pathway of descent.

chapter 13

BONE AND JOINTS

1. Prognosis of osteogenic sarcoma is:
   A) Excellent
   B) Good
   C) Poor
   D) Good if it occurs in young patients
2. Serum acid phosphatase elevated level is associated with:
   A) Osteogenesis imperfecta
   B) Osteopetrosis
   C) Osteitis fibrosa cystica
   D) All of the above
3. Giant cell lesion is:
   A) Osteoid osteoma
   B) Brown tumour of hyperthyroidism
   C) Exostosis
   D) Fibrous dysplasia
4. Most common site of aneurysmal bone cyst is:
   A) Long bones
   B) Mandible
   C) Clavicle
   D) Rib
5. Marble bone disease is also known as:
   A) Osteogenesis imperfecta
   B) Osteopetrosis
   C) Perthe's disease
   D) None
6. X bodies called Birbeck's granules are seen in:
   A) Granulomatous vasculitis
   B) Amyloidosis
   C) Langerhans cell granulomatosis
   D) Idiopathic pulmonary haemosiderosis
7. Albers-Schonberg disease is:
   A) Osteoporosis
   B) Osteomalacia
   C) Osteogenesis imperfecta
   D) Osteopetrosis
8. Most common site of eosinophilic granuloma is:
   A) Radius
   B) Femur
   C) Skull
   D) Lumbar vertebrae
9. Synonyms of Paget's disease is
   A) Osteitis fibrosa
   B) Osteitis proliference
   C) Osteitis deformans
   D) None of the above
10. Most common complication of rubella is:
    A) Polyarthritis
    B) Encephalitis
    C) Orchitis
    D) Thrombocytopaenia
11. Physaliferous cells characteristic of:
    A) Admantinoma
    B) Chordoma
    C) Ewing's tumour
    D) Multiple myeloma

12. Rheumatoid arthritis with splenomegaly, and leukopaenia is:
A) Still's disease
B) Felty's syndrome
C) Sjogren's syndrome
D) Reiter's syndrome

13. Histiocytosis X is seen in all except:
A) Hand Schuller Christian disease
B) Eosinophilic granuloma
C) Letterer-Siwe disease
D) Torres syndrome

14. Small cell tumour of bone does not include:
A) Ewing's sarcoma
B) Malignant lymphoma
C) Osteoblastoma
D) Metastatic neuroblastoma

15. In Ochronosis, there is an increased pigmentation of:
A) Skin
B) Cartilage
C) Nails
D) All of the above

16. Melon-seed bodies in joint fluid are characteristic of:
A) Rheumatoid arthritis
B) Tuberculous arthritis
C) Septic arthritis
D) None of the above

17. Osteosarcoma characteristically may develop in cases of:
A) Osteogenesis imperfecta
B) Acromegaly
C) Osteopetriosis
D) Osteitis deformans

18. Causes of pathological facture include which of the following?
A) Osteogenesis imperfecta
B) Osteopetrosis
C) Osteoporosis
D) All of the above

19. Woven bone is not seen in:
A) Osteosarcoma
B) Metastatic carcinoma
C) Paget's disease
D) Osteoporosis

20. Paget's disease transform into:
A) Osteogenic sarcoma
B) Chondrosarcoma
C) Fibrosarcoma
D) All of the above

21. Biphasic type of histology is seen in which tumour?
A) Rhabdomyosarcoma
B) Synovial cell sarcoma
C) Osteosarcoma
D) Neurofibroma

22. Lacunar skull most frequently associated with:
A) Diabetes mellitus
B) Posterior fossa tumour
C) Encephalocele
D) Arnold-Chairi syndrome

23. Bone tumour arising from epiphysis is:
A) Giant cell tumour
B) Chondromyxoid fibroma
C) Ewing's tumour
D) Osteogenic sarcoma

24. Radiological appearance of giant cell tumour is:
A) Sunray
B) Onion skin
C) Soap bubble
D) Moth eaten

25. Codman's triangle is most likely to be associated with:
A) Chondrosarcoma
B) Multiple myeloma
C) Osteomyelitis
D) Osteogenic sarcoma

26. Commonest benign bone tumour is:
A) Osteoma
B) Chondroma
C) Osteochondroma
D) Osteoblastoma

27. Following are indications that an osteochondroma has undergone sarcomatous change except:
A) Cartilage cap more than 2 cm
B) Pain and increase in size
C) Increase in calcification
D) Soft tissue mass

28. Most common primary neoplasm involving skeletal system is:
A) Lymphoma
B) Osteosarcoma
C) Fibrosarcoma
D) Multiple myeloma

29. The pathogenesis of traumatic bone cyst is/are
A) Mild trauma
B) Failure of organization of clot
C) Degeneration of clot
D) All of the above.

30. The commonest extraskeletal manifestations of fibrous dysplasia is:
A) Cutaneous pigmentation
B) Endocrine abnormalities
C) Myxomas
D) Gastrointestinal polyposis

31. The most common malignant change occurring in fibrous dysplasia is:
A) Osteosarcoma
B) Chondrosarcoma
C) Squamous cell carcinoma
D) Ewing's sarcoma

32. The most common primary lymphoma of bone histologically belongs to:
A) Follicular lymphoma
B) Diffuse large B cell lymphoma
C) Burkitt's lymphoma
D) T-cell lymphoma

33. Rice bodies are seen in except:
A) Rheumatoid arthritis
B) Tubercular arthritis
C) Psoriatic arthritis
D) Gout

34. Osteomyelitis of jaw is seen in:
A) Caffey's disease
B) Osteomalacia
C) Osteoporosis
D) Osteopoikilosis

35. Most common site of simple bone cyst is:
A) Femur
B) Humerus
C) Tibia
D) Radius

36. Chondrocalcinosis is seen in:
A) Gout
B) Pseudogout
C) Septic arthritis
D) Osteoarthritis

37. Most common site of TB spine is:
A) Cervical
B) Dorso-lumbar
C) Lumbosacral
D) Sacral

38. Triple deformity of knee joint seen in:
A) Tuberculosis
B) Trauma
C) Malignant tumour
D) Sarcoidosis

39. Wind sweep deformity is seen in:
A) Ankylosing spondylitis
B) Scurvy
C) Rheumatoid arthritis
D) Rickets

40. Sabre tibia is seen in:
A) Congenital syphilis
B) Rickets
C) Gonorrhoea
D) Renal osteodystrophy

41. Geographic skull is seen in:
A) Thalassaemia
B) Hand Schuller Christian disease
C) Hydrocephalus
D) Paget's disease

42. In Paget's disease X-ray skull shows:
A) Hair-on end appearance

B) Osteoporosis circumscripta
C) Pepper and salt appearance
D) Punched out lesions

43. Punched out lesions in skull is seen in:
A) Thalassaemia
B) Hand Schuller Christian disease
C) Multiple myeloma
D) Paget's disease

44. Common sites of bone metastasis except:
A) Pelvis
B) Ribs
C) Lower end of femur
D) Upper end of humerus

45. Sclerotic bone lesion is seen in all/E
A) Fluorosis
B) Osteopetriosis
C) Secondaries from prostate
D) Hyperparathyroidism

46. Onion layering is seen in:
A) Osteogenic sarcoma
B) Ewing's sarcoma
C) Synovial sarcoma
D) Chondrosarcoma

47. Calcification of intervertebral disc is seen in:
A) Fluorosis
B) Alkaptonuria
C) Pseudogout
D) Hyperparathyroidism

48. Osteoporosis caused by all/except
A) Sarcoidosis
B) Hyperparathyroidism
C) Old age
D) Steroid therapy

49. Bone tumour which is hormone dependent:
A) Chondrosarcoma
B) Ewing's tumour
C) Osteoid osteoma
D) Fibrous dysplasia

50. Complications of Paget's disease is:
A) Osteogenic sarcoma
B) Deafness
C) Heart failure
D) All of the above

51. Herbeden nodes are seen in:
A) Osteoarthritis
B) Rheumatoid arthritis
C) Rheumatic arthritis
D) Psoriatic arthritis

52. Commonest site of vertebral tuberculosis is:
A) Tibia
B) Radius
C) Humerus
D) Vertebrae

53. In Tietze's disease:
A) There is a small retromammary fibroadenoma
B) There is a swelling of second costal cartilage
C) The swelling should be explored
D) There is a painful swelling of second costal cartilage

54. Painless effusions in joints in congenital syphilis is called
A) Clutton's joints
B) Banton's joints
C) Charcot's joints
D) Synovitis

55. Ollier's disease refers to a condition characterized by:
A) Multiple osteochondroma
B) Multiple osteoid osteoma
C) Multiple enchondroma
D) Multiple exostosis

56. Osteolytic lesions of multiple myeloma are commonest in:
A) Femur
B) Pelvis
C) Clavicle
D) Vertebrae

57. A malignant tumour of childhood that metastasize to bone often is:
A) Wilm's tumour
B) Neuroblastoma
C) Adrenal gland tumour
D) Granulosa cell tumour

Answers

1. C) Osteogenic sarcoma is most aggressive tumour of children. 50% of cases of osteogenic sarcoma are at 60 years of age develops in pre-existing Paget's disease. The prognosis of osteogenic sarcoma is poor.

2. D) Serum acid phosphatase elevated level is seen in osteogenesis imperfecta, osteopetrosis and osteitis fibrosa cystica.

3. B) Brown tumour is a non-neoplastic lesion resulting from abnormal bone metabolism in hyperparathyroidism.

Histopathology shows network of ovoid to spindle shaped mesenchymal cells with focal aggregates of multinucleated giant cells diffusely present throughout the lesion.

Giant cell lesion of bone is brown tumour of hyperthyroidism. Other giant cell lesions of bone include: Osteoclastoma, solitary bone cyst, aneurysmal bone cyst, chondromyxoid fibroma, chondroblastoma, and ossifying fibroma.

4. A) Aneurysmal bone cyst occurs in lower leg (24%), upper extremity (21%), spine (16%), femur (13%), pelvis and sacrum (12%). Other sites include skull, mandible, clavicle, ribs and foot.

5. B) Osteopetrosis literally "stone bone" also known as marble bone disease extremely rare inherited disorder whereby the bone hardens, becoming denser. It is due to deficiency of carbonic anhydrase in osteoclasts is noted.

6. C) Birbeck's granules are rod shaped or tennis racket cytoplasmic organelles with a central linear density and a striated appearance. They are characteristic finding in Langerhan's cell granulomatosis (Histiocytosis X).

7. D) Albers-Schonberg disease is also known as osteopetrosis. This is an extremely rare inherited condition where bones harden becoming denser.

8. C) Eosinophilic granuloma is found in skull, mandible, spine, femur calvarium and ribs. Skull is most often affected (70-90%).

9. C) Paget's disease is also known as Osteitis deformans.

10. A) Up to 70% of adult women with rubella has pain, and/or swellings of the joints. A virus causes rubella. Complications of rubella include encephalitis, rash on face progresses down the body. Other complications include lymphadenopathy, orchitis, bronchitis, pneumonia, and thrombocytopaenia.

11. B) Physaliferous cells are characteristic cells in a tumour known as Chordoma. The chordoma consists of cords of epitheloid cells with eosinophilic cytoplasm in a mucinous stroma. The physaliferous cells are large cells with large vacuoles that displace the nucleus at the periphery. Immunohistochemical analysis reveals that the tumour cells are positive for S100 and cytokeratins and negative for calponin.

12. B) Felty's syndrome is defined by the presence of three conditions, rheumatoid arthritis, an enlarged spleen and abnormally low white blood cells. It affects less than 1% of patients with rheumatoid arthritis.

Still's disease is characterized by arthralgia, elevated serum ferritin, and salmon-pink rash, pyrexia and lymphadenopathy.

Reiter's syndrome is a rare disease characterized by arthritis, non-gonococcal urethritis, and conjunctivitis.

Sjogren's syndrome is a chronic autoimmune disorder characterized by xerostomia, xerophthalmia, and rheumatoid arthritis.

13. D) Histiocytosis X includes, eosinophilic granuloma, Letterer Siwe disease and Hand-Schuller-Christian disease. It is a variant of hereditary non-polyposis colorectal cancers. Muir Torre syndrome (MTS) is an inherited cancer disorder. Individuals are more prone to develop cancers of the colon, uterus, breast, genitourinary tract, stomach, ovarian, hepatobiliary and skin lesions, such as keratoacanthomas and sebaceous carcinoma. The genes affected are MLH 1 and MSH 2 and involved in DNA mismatch repair.

14. C) Osteoblastoma: Microscopically the intervening stroma is made up of loose vascular connective tissue instead of normal marrow elements and contains a large number of giant cells. Small cell tumours comprise of a diverse group of primary and metastatic neoplasms in both children and adults. The most common small cell tumours of bone include Ewing's sarcoma, neuroblastoma, lymphoma, leukaemia, rhabdomyosarcoma, and Langerhan cell histiocytosis.

15. D) Ochronosis, often called alkaptonuric ochronosis is an autosomal recessive metabolic disorder that causes an excess of homogentisic acid, resulting in adverse pigmentation, and inflammation of cartilaginous and related tissue throughout body. The clinical discolouration of the skin is a result of formation of ochronotic pigment granules in the dermis and in the apocrine glands. Ochronotic discolouration can also be detected on the nasal tip, the costochondral junctions, the extensor tendons of the hands, the cheeks, the fingernails, and the buccal mucosa.

The disease is characterized by blue-black pigmentation of the sclera, cartilage and synovial membranes as well as joint deterioration.

16. A) Melon–seed bodies are characteristic of rheumatoid arthritis. Radiologically there are "melon-seed" bodies due to inflammatous villus projection, which hang into the joint cavity from thickened synovial membrane.

17. D) In osteitis deformans the affected bone becomes cancerous in less than 1% of people. People whose disease progresses to bone cancer can develop an osteosarcoma, fibrosarcoma, or chondrosarcoma.

18. D) Non-neoplastic causes of pathological fracture include osteofibrous dysplasia, osteogenesis imperfecta, osteitis fibrosa cystica, osteoporosis, osteopetrosis, osteomalacia and osteomyelitis.

19. D) Woven bone: Bony tissue characteristic of the skeleton in which the collagen fibres of the matrix are arranged irregularly in the form of interlacing networks. Also called non-lamellar bone, reticulated bone. Osteoporosis is a disease of bone that leads to an increased risk of fracture. In osteoporosis the bone mineral density is reduced. Bone microarchitecture is disrupted.

20. D) Most common tumour arises from Paget's disease is osteosarcoma, followed by chondrosarcoma, fibrosarcoma, malignant fibrous histiocytoma, and reticulum cell sarcoma.

21. B) The synovial sarcoma consists of large polygonal cells (epitheloid) that secrete hyaluronic acid and show an organization that is suggestive of microscopic joint spaces. These cells are surrounded by spindle cells that simulate subsynovial mesenchymal cells.

It can be monophagic or biphagic.

Biphagic variant consists of plump round cells, and fibroblasts alternating with gland like areas that is lined by synovial like cells and contain mucin.

22. C) Lacunar skull is a congenital skull defect characterized by abnormal osseous, finger like impressions seen at the inner vault of the skull separated by dense bony ridges making a mesh-like structure on plain radiograph. Lacunar skull is always associated with encephalocele.

23. A) Bone tumour arising from epiphysis is giant cell tumour.

Chondromyxoid fibroma and osteogenic sarcoma arises from metaphysis, and Ewing's sarcoma from diaphysis.

24. C) On X-ray giant cell tumour of bone shows solitary expansile lytic lesion with multiple septation (soap bubble appearance). Sunray appearance is characteristic X-ray finding in osteogenic sarcoma. Radiologically Ewing's sarcoma is often associated with a lamellated or onion-skin periosteal reaction. The onion-skin appearance is followed with a moth eaten or mottled appearance.

25. D) Codman's triangle is a term used to describe the triangular area of new subperiosteal bone that is created when a lesion, often a tumour, raises the periosteum away from the bone. The main causes for this sign are osteosarcoma, Ewing's tumour and subperiosteal abscess. In Ewing's sarcoma the laminated appearance occurs towards the edge of the tumour where there may be Codman's triangle. There is usually a soft tissue mass rarely containing calcification.

26. C) Osteochondroma is one of the most common benign tumours of bone, accounting for approximately 35% of benign tumours.

Clinical features: The most common sites for osteochondroma are at the growing ends of bone, including the distal femur, proximal tibia, and proximal humerus.

Macroscopically: Osteochondroma vary in size, and larger lesions may project outward.

Microscopically: The histology shows a well-circumscribed lesion of mature lamellar bone or cartilage or a mixture of those tissues.

27. C) Indications that osteochondroma has undergone malignant change are:

1. Cartilage cap varies in considerably in thickness but is normally 2-3 mm in thickness. Secondary chondrosarcomas are usually at least 2 cm in thickness.
2. Cartilaginous cap in excess of one cm thickness or 5 cm in diameter are suggestive of malignancy.
3. Cortical destruction
4. Backgrowth of cartilaginous cap into the stalk or medullary canal.
5. Lysis of calcifications in cap.

28. B) Most common primary neoplasm involving skeletal system is osteogenic sarcoma.

29. D) The pathogenesis of simple bone cyst is unknown. Evidence exists that venous obstruction and blockage of interstitial fluid drainage, in an area of rapidly growing and remodeling cancellous bone, may play an important role in the formation of unicameral bone cysts. Other factors include failure of organization of clot, degeneration of clot, cystic degeneration of cysts and tumour, faulty calcium metabolism, ischemic necrosis, localized disturbances in bone and mild trauma.

30. A) Cutaneous pigmentation in polyostotic fibrous dysplasia is ipsilateral to the side of the bony lesions. Cutaneous pigmentation is the most common extraskeletal manifestation in fibrous dysplasia. It occurs in 50% of cases of the polyostotic form.

31. A) Sarcomatous changes occurring in fibrous dysplasia are osteosarcoma, chondrosarcoma, fibrosarcoma, and malignant fibrous histiosarcoma. The most common malignant change occurring in fibrous dysplasia is osteosarcoma.

32. B) Most common lymphoma that affects the bone is non-Hodgkin's lymphoma (NHL). Hodgkin's lymphoma is much less likely to be found. Among the different types of non-Hodgkin's lymphoma, diffuse large-B cell lymphoma (DLBL) is the most common.

33. D) Rice bodies are detached synovial villi lying within the joint cavity, which resemble grains of rice. These bodies vary in consistency, size and shape.

The majority of rice bodies are composed of coarsely reticulin material reacting immunologically with antifibrinogen, antireticulin, fibronectin and containing mononuclear cells.

Rice bodies are seen in:

1. Rheumatoid arthritis
2. Tuberculous arthritis
3. Agammaglobulinaemia
4. Hypogammaglobulinaemia
5. Psoriatic arthritis
6. Still's disease
7. Osteoarthritis
8. Ankylosing spondylitis
9. Juvenile rheumatoid arthritis
10. Seronegative inflammatory arthritis

34. A) CAFFEY-SILVERMAN SYNDROME: It is also known as Caffey's disease, Caffey's syndrome, and familial subperiosteal bone formation. It was first described in detail in 1945.

Clinical features: Infantile cortical hyperostosis is believed to exist in two forms, familial and sporadic.

Familial form seems to have an earlier onset; 24% of these cases occur at birth. Incidence of mandibular involvement is less than that observed in the sporadic form.

Sporadic form is becoming less common. It has a higher incidence of mandibular involvement than does the familial form.

Infantile cortical hyperostosis is a proliferative bone disease of infants under 6 months of age. The average age at time of diagnosis is 9 weeks.

Peculiar to this disease is bilateral subperiosteal new bone formation, most commonly involving mandible. Less commonly the clavicle, tibia, ulna, femur, ribs, humerus and fibula were involved with periodic proliferation in the first 3 months of life. The disease follows fever, usually appearing before 6 months of age and disappearing during childhood.

Oral manifestations

Puffy jaws and cheeks give the face a characteristic appearance. Enamel hypoplasia may be present.

Radiological findings: Typical radiologic feature is a marked periosteal new bone formation surrounding the diaphysis of long bones. The new bone becomes lamellated as the activity of the condition subsides and the bone becomes normal.

Histological findings:

1. Overlying periosteum shows inflammatory infiltrate.
2. The subperiosteal bone shows immature lamellar bone formation.

35. B) It usually occurs in the long bones of growing child especially the upper end of humerus (50 to 60 % of the time) or the upper part of femur (25 to 30% of the time). These cysts usually affect the children between 5 to 15 years, but can affect older children or adults.

The pathogenesis of simple bone cyst is unknown. Evidence exists that venous obstruction and blockage of interstitial fluid drainage, in an area of rapidly growing and remodeling cancellous bone, may play an important role in the formation of unicameral bone cysts.

PATHOLOGY

Macroscopically: On gross examination, the cyst expands the cortex of the bone. An instant periosteum covers this thin cortical shell. Simple bone cyst is a fluid filled cavity in the bone, lined by compressed fibrous tissue. Occasionally blood products may be found within the fluid if a previous fracture has occurred. A membrane of varying thickness lines the inner wall of the cyst. Fibrous septa may form after a fracture and create a multilocular appearance.

Microscopically: Mesothelial cells line simple bone cysts. The inner wall of bone adjacent to mesothelial membrane consists of well-vascularized new bone produced by the overlying periosteum. Multinucleated giant cells may be present within the cyst wall.

36. B) Pseudogout refers to the acute symptoms of joint inflammation or synovitis: red, tender, and swollen joints that may resemble gouty arthritis. Chondrocalcinosis on the other hand, refers to the radiographic evidence of calcification in hyaline and/or fibrocartilage. Pyrophosphate arthropathy is due to accumulation of crystals of calcium pyrophosphate dihydrate in the connective tissue. Knee joint is most commonly affected.

37. B) Pot's disease is a presentation of extrapulmonary tuberculosis that affects the spine, a kind of tuberculous arthritis of the intervertebral joints. It is named after Percivall Pott, a London Surgeon who trained at St Bartholomero's hospital, London. The lower thoracic and upper lumbar vertebrae are the areas of the spine most often affected. Scientifically, it is called tuberculous spondylitis and it is most commonly localized in the thoracic position of the spine.

Sign and symptoms include:
- Back pain
- Fever
- Night sweating
- Anorexia
- Weight loss

Spinal mass associated with numbness, paraesthesia, or muscle weakness of the legs.

Complications

Vertebral collapse resulting in kyphosis

Spinal cord compression

Sinus formation

Paraplegia (so called Pott's paraplegia)

38. A) Triple deformity of is seen in:
1. Tuberculosis
2. Polio
3. Rheumatoid arthritis
4. Rheumatic fever

Triple deformity of knee includes:
1. Flexion at the knee
2. Posterior subluxation of the tibia
3. External rotation of tibia (abduction) knee is common site for skeletal tuberculosis. It affects younger individuals. The patient presents with pain, stiffness, and deformity. The disease goes through stages of synovitis, arthitis, and fibrous ankylosis. Radiograph reveals triad of osteoporosis, joint space reduction erosions and destruction of bone.

39. D) Wind-sweep deformity is a skeletal seen in rickets. The term wind-sweep deformity describes the appearance of abnormal valgus deformity in one knee in association with varus deformity in the other.

40. A) Sabre tibia is a deformation of the tibia as a result of syphilis. It manifests as a forward convex shape created by gumma formation and periosteitis.

41. B) HAND SCHULLER CHRISTIAN DISEASE

A more localized variant, primarily referred to as Hand Schuller Christian disease, or multifocal eosinophilic granuloma is a childhood disease that consists of the triad of diabetes insipidus, lytic bone lesions and proptosis. It is the result of error of metabolism of cholesterol and its esters.

The age group involved is more than 3 years of age. It is more common in boys than girls 2:1.

X-ray skull shows confluent areas of destruction may isolate islands of bone, creating the geographic skull.

42. B) In the skull, the initial osteolytic phase of Paget's is called osteoporosis circumscripta due to the presence of geographic lucent regions primarily within frontal bone. This is followed by excessive new bone formation leading to cortical thickening and osteosclerotic changes in the inner table, diploae, and subsequently the inner surface of the outer table. In this phase, plain radiographs manifest a characteristic "cotton wool appearance of sclerotic lesions surrounded by areas of demineralization.

43. C) In cases of multiple myeloma, X-ray skull shows small-circumscribed areas of rarefaction of the bone (cannon ball). Bone changes consist of either diffuse decalcification or localized areas of bone destruction or a combination of two. Classically the lesions are seen as punched out defects in the bone.

44. C) Lower end of femur is not a site of bone metastasis.

Metastasis can occur in any bone in the body, but are found in bones near the center of the body. The spine is the most common site of bone metastasis.

Other common sites are the hip bone (pelvis), upper end of femur, upper end of humerus rib and the skull.

45. D) Hyperparathyroidism is an osteolytic lesion not osteosclerotic.

Sclerotic bone lesions are:

I. Vascular
 (a) Haemangiomas
 (b) Infarcts
II. Infection
 (a) Chronic osteomyelitis
III. Neoplasm
 (a) Primary
  (i) Osteoma
  (ii) Osteosarcoma
 (b) Metastatic
  (i) Prostate
  (ii) Breast
  (iii) Others
IV. Drugs
 (a) Vitamin D
 (b) Fluoride
V. Inflammatory/idiopathic
 (a) Congenital
  (i) Bone islands
  (ii) Osteopetrosis
  (iii) Pyknodysostosis
 (b) Autoimmune
 (c) Trauma
 Metabolic/endocrine
 Paget's disease

46. B) **Ewing's sarcoma: X-rays:** On conventional radiograph, the most common osseous presentation is a permeative lytic lesion with periosteal reaction. The classic description of lamellated or "*onion skin*" type of periosteal reaction is often associated with this lesion. Ewing's sarcoma is typically located in the medullary cavity and produces expansion of the affected diaphysis, often extending into the adjacent soft tissue. About 10 % presents with multiple bone involvement usually representing metastasis.

Chondrosarcoma: Radiologically: X-rays will show expansible lesion, thickening of cortex, and endosteal scalloping. Soft tissue mass may be seen along with characteristic punctate calcification within the bone.

Osteogenic sarcoma: X-ray shows bone destruction or new bone formation and characteristic sunray appearance.

47. B) In cases of alkaptonuria in the second and third decade the most distinctive finding is the laminated calcification of multiple intervertebral discs. Commonly all interspaces are affected and dramatically emphasized by the osteoporosis in the adjoining vertebrae.

Other causes of calcification of intervertebral disc is:

Ochronosis

CPPD crystal deposition disease

Acromegaly

Haemochromatosis

Hyperparathyroidism
Poliomyelitis
Amyloidosis
Spinal fusion

48. A) Osteoporosis is not seen in sarcoidosis.

Primary generalized osteoporosis is associated with aging.

Factors responsible for etiology of primary osteoporosis are as follows:

Hormonal factors (Postmenopausal): Hormonal factors play a significant role in the development of osteoporosis, especially in postmenopausal women. The bone loss associated with estrogen deficiency may be caused by a combination of increased bone resorption and decreased bone formation.

Senile: Senile osteoporosis occurs in adults of both sexes and increases in severity with age. Testosterone deficiency is present in about one third of men with senile osteoporosis.

Genetic: Certain variations of the vitamin D receptor gene are associated with a lower maximum bone density, presumably because they impair the bone forming effects of vitamin D.

Secondary generalized osteoporosis could be secondary to other known states or diseases.

Causes of secondary osteoporosis

(a) **Endocrine**: Hyperparathyroidism, hyperprolactinaemia, hyper-or hypothyroidism, ovarian or adrenal failure, pituitary tumours, insulin dependent diabetes mellitus and Cushing's syndrome.

(b) **Neoplasia**: Multiple myeloma, carcinomatosis, osteolytic metastases.

(c) **Gastro-intestinal diseases**: Malnutrition, malabsorption, vitamin C and D deficiencies, and chronic liver diseases.

(d) **Drug induced osteoporosis**: Corticosteroids, oral contraceptives, anticoagulants, chemotherapy, alcohol.

(e) **Mechanical factors**: Reduced physical activity is associated with accelerated bone loss.

(f) **Others**: Rheumatoid arthritis, psoriatic arthritis.

49. D) Fibrous dysplasia: Abnormality that occurs in the bone cells of fibrous dysplasia may also occur in the cells of some of the body's glands. This can lead to hormonal abnormalities. This is rare and generally happens with severe form of polyostotic fibrous dysplasis.

McCune-Albright syndrome is a condition where polyostotic fibrous dysplasia occurs with pigmented skin lesions (café-au-lait spots) and hormonal abnormalities.

Young patients may develop early puberty. This problem is more common in girls than boys. This is usually caused by overactivity of the ovaries. Overactivity may also occur in other glands of the body including:

1. Thyroid glands
2. Adrenal glands
3. Pituitary glands
4. Parathyroid glands

50. D) Complications of Paget's disease is:

Paget's disease may lead to other medical conditions including:

1. Osteogenic sarcoma
2. Arthritis
3. Loss of hearing
4. Cardiovascular disease can result from severe Paget's disease.
5. Kidney stones
6. Nervous system problems such as pressure on the brain, spinal cord or nerves
7. Loss of vision
8. When Paget's disease affects the facial bones the teeth may become loose. Disturbances in chewing may occur.

9. Angoid streaks may develop possibly as a result of calcification of collagen or other pathological deposition.

51. A) Osteoarthritis: Herbedens nodes are hard or bony swellings that can develop in distal interphalangeal joints (DIP) They are signs of osteoarthritis and caused by formation of osteophytes (calcific spurs) of the articular joint cartilage in response to repeated trauma at the joint.

52. D) Commonest site of tuberculosis is vertebrae.

53. B) Tietze's syndrome develop tenderness and swelling over the ribs and cartilage near the (breast bone) sternum. Redness, tenderness and heat can also be present but a localized swelling is distinguishing finding.

54. A) Clutton's joint is a term describing the finding of symmetrical joint swelling seen in patients with congenital syphilis. It most commonly affects the knees, presenting with synovitis, and joint effusions lasting up to a year. It has also been reported affecting the ankles, elbows, wrists, and fingers.

Charcot's joint refers to progressive degeneration of a weight bearing joint, a process marked by bony destruction, bone resorption and eventual deformity. Diabetes as well as peripheral neuropathy is the main risk factor for Charcot foot.

Other causes are:

1. Syphilis
2. Leprosy
3. Alcoholic neuropathy
4. Spinal cord injury
5. Cerebral palsy
6. Renal dialysis

55. C) Ollier's disease is a rare non-hereditary sporadic disorder where intraosseous benign cartilaginous tumour develops close to growth plate cartilage. Enchondromas are benign neoplasms of cartilage. In the bone, these can occur entirely within the bone (known as enchondromas). Nominally the disease consists of multiple enchondromas which usually develop in childhood.

56. D) Osteolytic lesions of multiple myeloma are commonest in vertebrae. The bones generally involved are those containing red bone marrow, e.g., vertebrae (66%), ribs (44%), skull (41%), pelvis (28%), femur (24%), clavicle (10%), scapula (10%).

57. B) Neuroblastoma is a tumour of childhood that metastasizes most often to bone.

chapter 14

MUSCLE AND NERVE PATHOLOGY

1. Progressive myositis ossificans results from mutation of gene?
   A) CLCN 1 gene
   B) GNAS 1 gene
   C) SCN4A gene
   D) NF-1 gene
2. Isaac's syndrome is:
   A) Acquired myotonia
   B) Congenital myotonia
   C) Dystrophic myotonia
   D) Paramyotonia
3. Myasthenia gravis is characterized by all except:
   A) Proximal muscle involvement
   B) Fatigue with exertion
   C) Spontaneous regression sometimes
   D) Absent deep reflexes
4. Which of the following is not a X- linked recessive muscular dystrophy?
   A) Duchenne's muscular dystrophy
   B) Becker's muscular dystrophy
   C) Limb-girdle muscular dystrophy
   D) Emery-Dreifuss muscular dystrophy
5. Periodic paralysis may be associated with all of the following except?
   A) Hyperkalaemia
   B) Hypokalaemia
   C) Hyperthyroidism
   D) Hypothyroidism
6. Myasthenia gravis is a disease of:
   A) Neuromuscular junction
   B) Neuromediators
   C) Neurons
   D) Muscle
7. Which of these is not a Congenital myopathy?
   A) Central core disease
   B) Nemaline dystrophy
   C) Central nuclear dystrophy
   D) Z-band myopathy
8. Claw hand is caused by lesion of:
   A) Ulnar nerve
   B) Median nerve
   C) Axillary nerve
   D) Radial nerve
9. Type I fibre atrophy is seen in muscle biopsy:
   A) Polio
   B) Myotonic dystrophy
   C) Myasthenia gravis
   D) Duchenne's syndrome
10. Serum creatinine kinase is elevated in all except:
    A) Becker's muscular dystrophy
    B) Acute polymyositis
    C) Central core myopathies
    D) Acute myoglobinic myopathy
11. Complications of Duchenne muscular dystrophy is:
    A) Cardiomyopathy

B) Pneumonia
C) Respiratory failure
D) All of the above

12. Death in myasthenia gravis is due to:
A) Cardiac failure
B) Depression of CNS
C) Respiratory failure
D) All of the above

13. Atrophy of muscles occurs in:
A) Degeneration
B) Vascular changes
C) Cachexia
D) All of the above

14. Characteristics of Subacute combined degeneration of spinal cord are all of the following except:
A) Cause deep sensory loss
B) Occurs only in vitamin B_{12} deficiency
C) Occur before anaemia
D) Caused by vascular mechanism

15. Parasite, which involves the striated muscle is:
A) Schistosomiasis
B) Trichinella spiralis
C) Filaria
D) Round worm

16. Myositis ossificans is commonly seen in:
A) Knee
B) Elbow
C) Shoulder
D) Hip

17. Characteristic finding in muscular dystrophy is:
A) Inflammatory cell infiltrate
B) Heterogenicity of fibre size
C) Nuclear proliferation
D) Muscle necrosis

Answers

1. B) Multicentric myositis ossificans also known as progressive osseous heteroplasia results from mutations of GNAS-1 gene. Progressive osseous heteroplasia (POH) is a recently described genetic disorder of mesenchymal differentiation characterized by dermal ossification during infancy and progressive heterotopic ossification of cutaneous subcutaneous and deep connective tissues during childhood.

2. A) Issac's syndrome is a rare disorder with onset usually in late childhood or early childhood characterized by intermittent or continuous widespread involuntary muscle contractions, fasciculation, hyporeflexia, muscle cramp, muscle weakness, hyperhydrosis, tachycardia. The continuous motor actively persists during sleep and general anaesthesia. Familial and acquired (primary autoimmune) forms have been reported.

3. D) In cases of myasthenia gravis sensations and deep reflexes are normal. Other characteristics of myasthenia gravis include proximal muscle involvement. There is weakness of muscles. Myasthenia gravis involves episodic muscle weakness, and easy fatigability. Weaknesses resolve when the affected muscles are rested but recur when they are used again.

4. C) Sex linked muscular dystrophies include Duchenne muscular dystrophy, Becker's muscular dystrophy, and Emery-Dreifuss muscular dystrophy. Limb girdle muscular dystrophy has autosomal recessive or dominant type of inheritance.

5. D) Periodic paralysis is an autosomal dominant myopathy with considerable variation in penetrance, leading to a spectrum of familial phenotypes (only one parent needs to carry the gene mutation to affect the children but not all family members) who share the gene are affected to the same degree. Periodic paralysis occurs in hypokalemia, hyperkalemia, hyperparathyroidism, and hyperthyroidism. Hypothyroidism is not included under periodic paralysis disease.

6. A) Myasthenia gravis is a neuromuscular disease leading to fluctuating muscle weakness and fatigability. It is an autoimmune disorder, in which muscle circulating antibodies that block acetylcholine receptors at the post-synaptic neuromuscular junction causes weakness.

7. D) The conditions included under the term congenital myopathy are nemaline myopathy, myotubular myopathy, central core myopathy, congenital fibre type disproportion, muticore myopathy and core rod myopathy.

8. A) Ulnar nerve injuries commonly occur where nerve passes posterior to the medial condyle of humerus. Ulnar nerve injury patients have difficulty in making a fist because they cannot flex 4th and 5th digits at the distal interphalangeal joints. This characteristic appearance of the hand resulting from a distal lesion of the ulnar nerve is known as claw hand.

9. B) Muscle biopsy in myotonic dystrophy shows rows of internal nuclei, ring fibres sarcoplasmic masses, type 1 fibre atrophy and a greatly increased number of intrafusal muscle fibres.

10. D) Causes of increased creatinine kinase in muscle diseases.

Dystrophy

Dystrophinopathy
Myotonic dystrophy
Limb – Girdle muscular dystrophy
Fascio – Scapulo humeral dystrophy
Oculo – Pharyngeal muscular dystrophy

Metabolic

Glycogen storage disorders
GPT_2 deficiency
AMPDA deficiency

Other hereditary myopathy

Central core
Myotonic dyst
Backer muscular dystrophy
Danon
Distal
Malignant hypothermia
Mitochondrial disease
Myofibrillar myopathy
Myopathy with tubular aggregates
Myotonia congenita DM_2
Rippling muscle syndromes

Acquired disorders

Inflammatory – Acute polymyositis, viral myositis
Drug toxicity
Degeneration – Motor neuron diseases, but not polyneuropathies

Idiopathic

Hereditary idiopathic

Others

Exercise, traffic accidents, intramuscular injections, surgery

11. D) Complications of Duchenne's muscular dystrophy include cardiomyopathy, pneumonia, and respiratory failure. Other complications are congestive cardiac failure, mental impairment and scoliosis.

12. C) More severe myasthenia gravis affects multiple muscular regions and may be sufficiently severe to cause respiratory failure and death if untreated. Pneumonia is a common complication in patients with myasthenia gravis and often causes death in fatal cases.

13. D) Muscle atrophy is defined as a decrease in the cell mass of muscle. Muscle atrophy occurs in cachexia, vascular changes (poor circulation), amyotrophic lateral sclerosis, Gullain-Barre syndrome, poliomyelitis, injury, diabetic neuropathy, osteoarthritis, starvation, and stroke. Electron microscopic observations on "hyaline degeneration: of skeletal muscles occurring in a patient with severe muscle atrophy due to hypertrophic neuritis".

14. D) Subacute combined degeneration of the spinal cord is a result of vitamin B_{12} deficiency. Lack of this vitamin is often caused by pernicious anaemia or vitamin B_{12} disorder that prevents absorption of vitamin B_{12}. Most often anaemia symptoms are the most common symptoms of the disorder, but subacute combined degeneration can occur without those symptoms. The symptoms of subacute combined degeneration include tingling and numbness. Weakness of the legs, arms, trunk, changes in mental states. It is thought that lack of vitamin causes an abnormal formation of fatty acids, which are used by the body to build cell membranes and the nerve myelin sheath.

15. B) The parasite, which can be detected histologically in striated muscle is trichinella spiralis. The clinical effects depend on the intensity of infections: 90% of infections are light, but symptoms usually develop when there are more than 10 larvae per gram of skeletal muscle: they include the clinical picture of acute myalgia, edema, and fever.

16. B. Elbow

Myositis ossificans circumscripta is commonly caused by local trauma and is common as sports injury in the contact setting. The lesion occurs 80% of the time in arm (wrist joint, biceps brachialis) but also occur in the thigh.

17. D) The histology picture of muscular dystrophy and typically with small clusters of necrotic fibres found at the periphery of the muscle fascicle.

chapter 15

Nervous System

1. Which is not a feature of extramedullary tumour?
   A) Early corticospinal and descending
   B) Root pain or middle back pain
   C) CSF normal
   D) Sacral sparing
2. Lacunar skull most frequently associated with:
   A) Diabetes mellitus
   B) Posterior fossa tumour
   C) Encephalocele
   D) Arnold-Chairi syndrome
3. Best prognostic cerebral tumour in children:
   A) Medulloblastoma
   B) Astrocytoma
   C) Glioma
   D) Meningioma
4. Psammoma bodies are characteristic of which of the following tumours?
   A) Astrocytoma
   B) Meningioma
   C) Ependymoma
   D) Neuroblastoma
5. Most common viral disease that can cause mental retardation in humans:
   A) Cytomegalovirus
   B) Herpes simplex
   C) Rubella
   D) Endemic parotitis
6. Negri body is most commonly seen in:
   A) Hippocampus
   B) Basal ganglion
   C) Mid brain
   D) Parietal cortex
7. Basal ganglia calcification is seen in except:
   A) Birth anoxia paralysis
   B) Hyperparathyroidism
   C) Wilson's disease
   D) Mitochondrial cytopathy
8. Most common location of hypertensive intracranial haemorrhage is:
   A) Subarachnoid space
   B) Basal ganglion
   C) Cerebellum
   D) Brain stem
9. Which of the following is not a primitive neuroectodermal tumour:
   A) Neuroblastoma
   B) Glioblastoma
   C) Medulloblastoma
   D) All of the above
10. Wernicke's encephalopathy is characterized by:
    A) Neck stiffness
    B) Ophthalmoplegia
    C) Grandmal epilepsy
    D) All of the above
11. Hirano bodies are characteristically seen in:
    A) Parkinson's disease
    B) Alzheimer's disease

C) Rabies
D) Kuru

12. Lewy bodies are seen in:
A) Parkinson's disease
B) Alzheimer's disease
C) Multiple system atrophy
D) All of the above

13. Following are the features of Alzheimer's disease except:
A) Hirano bodies
B) Neuritic plaques
C) Neurofibrillary tangles
D) Loss of pigment in substantia nigra

14. Which type of necrosis occurs following cerebral infarction:
A) Coagulation
B) Liquefaction
C) Caseous
D) Fat necrosis

15. Basal ganglia is not affected in:
A) Amyloid angiopathy
B) Fahr's syndrome
C) Co poisoning
D) Hypertensive haemorrhage

16. Characteristic feature of rabies is:
A) Brain stem encephalitis
B) Meningitis
C) Ventriculitis
D) Periarticular cuffing

17. Gitter cells are
A) Ependycytes
B) Oligodendrocytes
C) Astrocytes
D) Modified CNS macrophages

18. Nucleus involvement in Alzheimer's disease is:
A) Basal nucleus of Mayernet
B) Raphae nucleus
C) Superior salivary nucleus
D) Basal lobe of cerebellum

19. The most common site of brain abscess:
A) Frontal lobe
B) Parietal lobe
C) Occipital lobe
D) Temporal lobe

20. X-ray finding in cases of raised intracranial pressure is:
A) Silver beaten skull
B) Rice grain calcification
C) Hair on end appearance
D) Punched out areas

21. J shaped sella turcica is seen in:
A) Hydrocephalus
B) Hand-Schuller-Christian disease
C) Chromophobe adenoma
D) Empty sella syndrome

22. Rail road calcification involving the cerebral cortex is a feature of:
A) Glioblastoma multiformae
B) Sturge-Weber syndrome
C) Craniopharyngioma
D) Germ cell tumours

23. Suprasellar calcification is hall mark of:
A) Craniopharyngioma
B) Sturge-Weber syndrome
C) Meningioma
D) Tuberculosis

24. Intracranial brain tumour in children under 5 years include all/except:
A) Glioblastoma multiformae
B) Optic nerve glioma
C) Brain stem glioma
D) Medulloblastoma

25. Suprasellar cystic mass in children is:
A) Medulloblastoma
B) Meningioma
C) Secondaries
D) Craniopharyngioma

26. The most common posterior fossa tumour in children is:
A) Astrocytoma
B) Medulloblastoma
C) Oligodendroglioma
D) Ependymoma

27. Most common childhood brain tumour is:
    A) Astrocytoma
    B) Medulloblastoma
    C) Oligodendroglioma
    D) Meningioma
28. Spinal cord compression may be caused by:
    A) Cysticercosis
    B) Ankylostomiasis
    C) Ecchinococcus-granulosus
    D) Visceral larva migrans
29. All are features of Wilson's disease Except:
    A) Increased copper content in liver
    B) Increased ceruloplasmin
    C) Mental changes
    D) Features of chronic active hepatitis
30. Periventricular calcification is often due to:
    A) Toxoplasmosis
    B) CMV
    C) Congenital syphilis
    D) All of the above
31. Metastasis outside the brain occur in this brain tumour:
    A) Craniopharyngioma
    B) Glioblastoma
    C) Medulloblastoma
    D) Haemangioblastoma

Answers

1. D) Extramedullary tumour may be inside the dura matter or outside the dura matter. In cases of extramedullary tumours there is no sacral sparing. Sacral sparing indicates a complete spinal cord injury where no motor or sensory function is preserved in the sacral segments S4-S5. The tumours can disseminate in CSF pathways. Back and progressive neurological symptoms are common. Patients have corticospinal and descending paralysis.

2. C) Lacunar skull refers to a characteristic radiograph appearance of the calvarium seen at birth with multiple focal areas of bone thinning, resembling a "copper beaten pattern". The condition is seen in children with encephalocele.

3. B) Most cerebellar astrocytomas are low grade pilocytic astrocytoma. However of all childhood tumours cerebellar astrocytoma have the best prognosis. Childhood low-grade astrocytomas have an excellent cure rate by tumour surgery alone.

4. B) Meningiomas are the second most common primary tumour of the central nervous system, arising from the arachnoid "cap" cells of the arachnoid villi in the meninges. Meningioma that contains psammoma bodies (from the Greek word Psammoma sand) i.e., concentric lamina of calcium salts in great profusion. Psammomatous calcifications aggregate into whorls and lobules with meningoepithelial cells. Psammoma bodies typically occur in meningoepitheliomatous or syncytial meningioma.

5. A) Congenital CMV infections is the most common cause of virus-induced mental retardation in Western World.

6. A) Negri bodies are eosinophilic, sharply outlined, pathognomonic inclusion bodies (2 to 10 μm in diameter) found in cytoplasm of certain nerve cells containing virus of rabies, especially in Ammon's horn of hippocampus.

7. A) Familial idiopathic basal ganglia calcification is a neurodegenerative disorder with characteristic calcium deposits in the basal ganglia. Other causes include metabolic diseases, hypothyroidism, mitochondrial cytopathy, toxoplasmosis, tuberculosis, pseudohypoparathyroidism, secondary hyperparathyroidism, (in renal disease), idiopathic cerebrovascular ferrocalcinosis, Cockayne syndrome, and Wilson's disease.

8. B) The area in which hypertensive haemorrhages most commonly occur is the basal ganglia. Other sites include thalamus, and cerebellum.

9. B) Glioblastoma is not a primitive ectodermal tumour. Primitive ectodermal tumours include neuroblastoma, medulloblastoma, Ewing's tumour, pineoblastoma, and melanotic neuroectodermal tumour of infancy.

10. B) Wernicke's encephalopathy is a syndrome characterized by ophthalmoplegia, grandmal epilepsy, ataxia, confusion and short term memory. It is caused by deficiency of thiamine (vitamin B_1) deficiency.

11. B) Hirano bodies are intracellular aggregates of actin, and actin associated proteins observed in the neurons of individuals affected with certain neurological disorders such as Alzheimer's disease as Creutzfeldt-Jacob disease. They are described as rod shaped crystal like and eosinophilic staining with haematoxylin and eosin. They are seen in hippocampal pyramidal cells.

12. D) **Lewy** bodies are abnormal aggregates of protein that develops inside nerve cells in Parkinson's disease. Lewy bodies are spherical masses that displace other cell components. There are two morphological types: Classical (brain stem) Lewy bodies and cortical Lewy bodies. A classical Lewy bodies is an eosinophilic cytoplasmic inclusion that consists of a dense core surrounded by halo of 10 nm wide radiating fibrils, the primary structural component of which is alpha granules. Lewy bodies are seen in Parkinson's disease, Alzheimer's disease, multiple system atrophy, dementia with Lewy bodies, Pick's disease and corticobasal degeneration.

13. D) Hirano bodies, neuritic plaques, and neurofibrillary tangles and Lewy bodies are features of Alzheimer's disease. In Parkinson's disease there is loss of pigmentation in the substantia nigra.

14. B) Liquefaction necrosis occurs following cerebral infarction. It is seen in the tissue containing excess of lipid and usually encountered in brain, which is as a result of ischaemic necrosis under going softening and rapid enzymatic autodigestion followed by liquefaction and cavity formation.

Macroscopically the tissue in the area of necrosis is liquefied and may be watery, tenacious or semisolid in consistency. The colour is white, yellow and red, if the necrosis is of long duration a connective tissue wall may be formed surrounding the necrotic tissue.

Microscopically: No architectural or cellular detail is visible in the area of necrosis. The dead tissue is homogenous and stains pink with eosin. In abscess, in neutrophils varying degrees of disintegration are found. Necrotic tissue in the central nervous system does not contain neutrophils.

15. A) Cerebral amyloid angiopathy refers to the deposition of B-amyloid in the media, an adventitia of small and midium-sized arteries of the cerebral arteries or cortex and leptomeninges. Fahr's disease, Co poisoning and hypertensive haemorrhage causes involvement of basal ganglia. Other causes of basal ganglia involvement occurs in attention-deficit hyperactivity disorder, cerebral palsy, dystonia, Huntington's disease, Lesch-Nyhan syndrome, Parkinson's disease, Tourette's disorder, Wilson's disease and blepharospasm. Fahr's disease is idiopathic basal ganglia calcification is a rarely genetically dominant inherited neurological disorder characterized by abnormal deposits of calcium in areas of the brain that control movement, including basal ganglia.

16. A) Always fatal encephalitis that is caused by the rabies virus is characterized by intense edema, vascular damage, necrosis, neuronal degeneration and inflammation with a predilection to the basal ganglia, midbrain, floor of the fourth ventricle, and the anterior motor neurons of the spinal cord.

17. D) Gitter cell or hortaga cell is a microglial cell that is globular and swollen after having phagocytized debris from cells destroyed pathologically in the central nervous system. Also called compound granule cell or compound granular corpuscle.

18. A) Nucleus basilis of Meynert, abbreviated NMB and also known as the nucleus basalis is a group of neurons in the substantia innominata of the basal forebrain which has wide projections to the neocortex and is rich in acetylcholine and choline acetyltransferase. In Alzheimer's disease nucleus undergoes degeneration. A decrease in acetylcholine production is seen in Alzeimer's disease.

19. A) The common sites of brain abscess are the white matter of frontal lobe, the parietal lobe and cerebellum. The commonest sources are the paranasal sinuses, a pulp space infection in a tooth, mastoiditis, infective endocarditis, congenital heart disease especially septal defects, lung abscesses, bronchiectasis, osteomyelitis in a distant bone, etc.

The causative organisms include the common pyogenic cocci and many others- anaerobic streptococci, diphtheroids and coliform etc.

20. A) Silver beaten skull (also known as beaten brass skull or copper beaten skull refers to the prominence of convoluted markings (gyral impressions on the inner table of the skull) seen through the skull vault. Underlying cause is thought to be related to increased intracranial pressure resulting from such processes as craniosynostosis, obstructive hydrocephalus, and/or intracranial masses.

21. D) J shaped sella: A term referring to the appearance of the sella turcica, which extends under anterior clinoid process and looks like a 'J' on its side. It may be rarely seen in normal adult skulls, but is a slightly more common in children (incidence of 5 to 6%). While it can be a normal anatomic variant, it may be associated with chronic hydrocephalus, raised intracranial pressure, gargoylism, Morquio's syndrome, Hurler's syndrome and other mucopolysaccharidoses as well as glioma of optic chiasma and empty sella syndrome.

X-ray skull shows elongated or boot-shaped sella turcica with an elongated anterior clinoid process.

Empty sella syndrome is a radiological finding where spinal fluid is found within the space created for the pituitary.

22. B) Rail road track or tram track calcification is seen in Sturge-Weber syndrome. There is curvilinear and double contour calcification of damaged cortical layer. Railroad track or tram track calcification is pathognomic in a child with facial nevus.

23. A) Suprasellar calcification is said to be the hallmark of a craniophyrngioma and occurs overall in more than 70% of tumours and nearby all the pediatric tumours.

Plain radiographs may reveal suprasellar calcifications, which are variable in appearance from thin "egg shell" plaques to dense solid popcorn calcifications. Calcifications are rarely off the midline to any significant degree.

Causes of intracranial calcification

I. Tumours: Glioma, craniopharyngioma, meningioma, ependymoma, chordoma, pinealoma, dermoid, lipoma, hamartoma, pituitary adenoma

II. Vascular: Arteriosclerosis, aneurysm, angioma, old haematoma

III. Infection and infestation: Tuberculosis, toxoplasmosis,

Cytomegalic inclusion, cysticercosis, paragonimiasis, old abscess

IV. Metabolic, miscellaneous: Idiopathic basal ganglia, hypothyroidism,

Pseudohyperparathyroidism, tuberous sclerosis,

Sturge-Weber, choroids plexus dystrophic calcification.

24. A) Intracranial tumours in childhood

Gliomas: Cerebellar gliomas, cerebral gliomas, astrocytoma, brain stem gliomas, ependymomas, optic nerve gliomas

Primitive neuroectodermal tumours: medulloblastoma,

Craniopharyngioma,

Pineal blastoma

Choroid plexus papilloma

Teratomas

Meningiomas

Ganglioglioma

25. D) Suprasellar cystic mass in children is craniopharyngioma. Craniopharyngioma is a slow growing, extra-axial, epithelial-squamous, calcified, cystic tumour arising from the remnants of the craniopharyngeal duct/ or Rathke cleft and occupying the supra sellar region.

26. A) Posterior fossa tumours are more common in children than in adults. Between 54 to 74% of all childhood brain tumours originate in posterior fossa.

Pilocytic astrocytoma is most common tumour in posterior fossa in children.

Posterior fossa masses include:

1. Pilocytic astrocytoma
2. Brain stem glioma
3. Medulloblastoma
4. Ependymoma
5. Atypical teratoid/rhabdoid tumour
6. Haemangioblastoma
7. Teratoma

27. B) Most common brain tumour is medulloblastoma.

28. C) Hydatid disease of spine is caused by the parasite echinococcus granulosus, a helminth belonging to the cestode group. Hydatidosis of bone occurs in 0.5-3% of all the cases. The vertebral column is involved in 50% of these. The disease usually spreads to the spine by direct extradural hydatid disease without any systemic foci are extremely rare. The sites affected are thoracic spine in 50%, lumbar spine in 20% and sacral spine in 20%.

29. B) The levels of ceruloplasmin are abnormally low (< less 0.2 g/L) in 80-95% of cases.

Wilson's disease or hepatolenticular degeneration is an autosomal recessive genetic disorder in which copper accumulates in tissue; this manifests as neurological or psychiatric symptoms and liver disease.

Chronic active hepatitis has caused cirrhosis of the liver in most by the time they develop symptoms.

The main sites of copper accumulation are the liver disease and the brain, and consequently liver disease and neuropsychiatric symptoms are the main features that lead to diagnosis.

30. B) CMV: Severe intrauterine brain infection, often with microcephaly and characteristic wide spread periventricular calcification may outline the dilated ventricle.

Toxoplasmosis: Calcification in congenital toxoplasmosis is characteristically consisting of scattered flecks in cortex and linear streaks in the basal ganglion.

31. C) Medulloblastoma is a highly malignant brain tumour that originates in the cerebellum or posterior fossa.

Medulloblastoma spread through the CSF and frequently metastasize to different locations in the brain and spine.

chapter 16

SKIN DISEASES

1. Severe bullous form of erythema multiforme is known as?
   A) Plummer-Vinson's syndrome
   B) Peutz-Jegher's syndrome
   C) Gardener's syndrome
   D) Stevens-Jonhson syndrome
2. Mutations in KRT14 and KRT5 genes causes:
   A) Lichen planus
   B) Epidermolysis bullosa
   C) Psoriasis
   D) Erythema multiforme
3. CREST variant of scleroderma is characterized by:
   A) Calcinosis
   B) Raynaud's phenomenon
   C) Esophageal dysfunction
   D) All of the above
4. Cerumoral pigmentation in the form of small melanotic spot is usually seen in:
   A) Plummer-Vinson's syndrome
   B) Lichen planus
   C) Erythema multiforme
   D) Peutz-Jegher's syndrome
5. Acanthosis is found in:
   A) Stratum spinosum
   B) Stratum lucidum
   C) Stratum corneum
   D) Basal cell layer
6. Following conditions are not associated with increased risk of malignancy except:
   A) Acanthosis nigricans
   B) Squamous papilloma
   C) Solar keratosis
   D) Erythema multiforme
7. Herald patch is commonly seen with:
   A) Pityriasis rosea
   B) Pityriasis versicolor
   C) Erysipelas
   D) Dermatophytosis
8. Contact allergy is associated with:
   A) Anaphylactoid reaction
   B) IgE mediated immunity
   C) Cell mediated immunity
   D) Immune complex disease
9. Erythema nodosum leprosum occurs in:
   A) Lepromatous leprosy
   B) Tuberculoid leprosy
   C) Both
   D) None
10. Indirect immunofluorescence test is done for the diagnosis of:
    A) Pemphigus
    B) Lichen planus
    C) Erythema multiforme
    D) Lupus erythematosus
11. Herald test is diagnostic of
    A) Pityriasis alba

B) Pityriasis rosea
C) Pityriasis rubra pilaris
D) Pityriasis versicolor

12. Which of the following does not predispose to squamous cell carcinoma?
A) Solar keratosis
B) Bowen's disease
C) Chronic eczema
D) Chronic ulceration

13. Commonest nerve involved in leprosy is:
A) Ulnar
B) Median
C) Radial
D) Musculocutaneous

14. Lesion not seen in lepromatous leprosy is:
A) Macule
B) Papule
C) Nodule
D) Vesicle

15. Which of the following condition arises from sweat gland?
A) Trichoepithelioma
B) Trichilemmoma
C) Clear cell hydradenoma
D) Trichefollicularis

16. Causes of erythema nodosum include:
A) Sarcoidosis
B) Tuberculosis
C) Inflammatory bowel disease
D) All of the above

17. Scl-70 antibody is characteristic of:
A) Systemic lupus erythematosus
B) Scleroderma
C) Dermatomyositis
D) Sjogren's syndrome

18. Drug induced lupus can be identified by:
A) Anti-histone antibodies
B) Double stranded DNA antibodies
C) Antinuclear antibodies
D) Anti-Sm antibodies

19. Skin peeling occurs in the following conditions except:
A) Infectious mononucleosis
B) Kawasaki disease
C) Scarlet fever
D) Toxic shock syndrome

20. Causes of leg ulcers:
A) Leprosy
B) Sickle cell anaemia
C) Diabetes mellitus
D) All of the above

21. Brooke's tumour is a tumour of:
A) Superficial dermal vessels
B) Sweat glands
C) Hair follicles
D) Sebaceous glands

22. Dermatophytes cause infection of:
A) Non-hairy skin
B) Hair
C) Nails
D) All of the above

23. All of the following are bacterial infections except:
A) Impetigo
B) Erysipelas
C) Furuncles
D) Kerion

24. Skin appendages include all of the following except:
A) Sebaceous gland
B) Eccrine sweat glands
C) Melanocytes
D) Apocrine sweat glands

25. Verruca vulgaris is:
A) Genital warts
B) Plantar warts
C) Common warts
D) Plane warts

26. Other name for basal cell papilloma is:
A) Molluscum contagiosum
B) Seborrhoeic keratosis
C) Clear cell carcinoma
D) Solar keratosis

27. Primary lesion of molluscum contagiosum is:
A) Macule
B) Papule

59. Cock peculiar tumour is synonyms:
   A) Rodent ulcer of nose
   B) Local osteomyelitis of the cranium
   C) Chronic infection of the sebaceous cyst
   D) Cylindroma
60. Marjolin's ulcer is:
   A) Squamous cell carcinoma from scar
   B) Adenoma of scar
   C) Tuberculous ulcer
   D) Basal cell carcinoma
61. Primary basal cell carcinoma occurs on:
   A) Skin and mucosa
   B) Skin and its pilosebaceous adnexa
   C) Skin, lip, and tongue
   D) All of the above
62. Skin smear is positive in all except:
   A) Maduramycosis
   B) Blastomycosis
   C) Cryptococcus
   D) Tinea versicolor

Answers

1. D) Stevens-Johnson syndrome, also called erythema multiforme major, is a symmetric, severe vesico-bullous eruption on at least two mucus membranes (oral, anorectal, and ocular membranes, lips) with frequent atypical target lesions affecting in some cases up to 15% of the body surface area.

2. B) Mutations in the KRT14 and KRT5 genes cause epidermolysis bullosa simplex.

Clinical features: Epidermolysis bullosa simplex is one of the major forms of epidermolysis bullosa. Blistering may primarily affect the hands and feet in milder cases, and the blisters usually heal without leaving scars. Severe cases of this condition involve widespread blistering that can lead to infection, dehydration, and other medical problems. Severe cases may be life threatening in infancy.

3. D) CREST variant form of scleroderma is milder disease than generalized scleroderma. Calcinosis, Raynaud's phenomenon, esophageal dysfunction, sclerodactly and telangiectasia characterize it.

4. D) Peutz-Jegher's syndrome is an autosomal dominant inherited disorder characterized by intestinal hamartomatous polyps in association with mucocutaneous melanotic macules. Mucocutaneous pigmentation and melanin spots are typical of patients with Peutz-Jegher's syndrome, and they are present in more than 95% of cases. They appear as small brown or dark blue spots with appearance of freckles most commonly in the peribuccal area. Cutaneous pigmentation (1-to-5 mm macules) is usually located in the perioral region, crossing the vermilion border (94%) in the paranasal and perioral area.

5. A) Acanthosis is diffuse epidermal hyperplasia. Acanthosis implies increased in stratum spinosum.

6. C) Solar keratosis results from sun damage and a small proportion can progress to malignancy. It is a premalignant condition of thick, scaly patches of skin.

7. A) Pityriasis rosea is a common benign skin disease, or exanthem, that was classified as a papulosquamous disorder, which means that the lesions are marked by small raised areas (papules) as well as scaly areas. Pityriasis rosea begins in 60 to 90% of patients with a pinkish-brown or salmon.

Coloured herald patch sometimes called mother patch on the chest, back, or neck. Herald patch is a small spot, when it first appears but enlarges over a period of several days to form a circular or oval shaped area between ¾ inch and 2½ inch in diameter.

8. C) Contact allergy results from a specific acquired hypersensitivity of the delayed type, also known as cell-mediated hypersensitivity (type IV) allergy or cell mediated immunity. For sensitization individuals must have significant and normally repeated contact with allergen. Therefore individuals may be exposed to allergens few years before finally developing hypersensitivity.

9. A) Erythema nodosum leprosum (ENL) is an immune-mediated complication of lepromatous leprosy presenting with inflammatory skin nodules. Immune complex production and as well as complementation have long been regarded as the principle etiology in ENL. ENL is characterized by an inflammatory infiltrate of neutrophils with vasculitis.

10. D) Antinuclear antibodies (ANAs) are directed against several nuclear antigens. Standard test for ANA is in assessing SLE because it is positive in close to 100% of patients with active SLE. Several techniques are used to detect ANAs. The most commonly used method is indirect immunoflourescence, which detects variety of nuclear antigens including RNA, and proteins.

11. B) Herald patch is seen in 80% of patients with pityriasis rosea. Oval, slightly raised plaque 2 to 5 cm, salmon-red, fine collarette scale at periphery; may be multiple. Pityriasis rosea is a skin rash that usually begins as one large, circular or oval spot on chest, abdomen or back. Called a herald patch, this initial spot can be 4 inches (10 cm) across.

12. C) Bowen's disease (also known as squamous cell carcinoma in situ) is a neoplastic skin disease. It can be considered as an early stage or intradermal form of squamous cell carcinoma. Causes of Bowen's disease include solar damage, arsenic, immunosuppression, viral infection, (human papilloma virus, or HPV) and chronic skin injury and dermatoses.

Actinic keratosis (also called "solar keratosis) is a premalignant condition of thick, scaly or crusty patches of skin. It progresses to squamous cell carcinoma. Squamous cell carcinoma can be a complication of chronic ulcers.

13. A) Commonest nerve involved in tuberculoid leprosy is ulnar nerve. Claw hand deformity usually indicative of ulnar nerve is most common in leprosy followed by median nerve; radial nerve involvement usually occurs with involvement of the above nerves

14. D) In lepromatous leprosy the skin lesions are multiple, slightly hypopigmented, erythematous macules, papules, nodules, and diffuse infiltration.

15. C) Clear cell hydradenoma is benign skin appendages (eccrine duct tumour). Histologically it contains small ductular lumens, focal apocrine and squamoid change, and a less prominent vascular pattern. They are usually circumscribed, non-capsulated tumours composed of polyhedral or fusiform cells with clear or eosinophilic cytoplasm. Trichilemmoma is a benign tumour neoplasm with pilosebaceous follicular epithelium. Trichoepitheliomas represents an uncommon hamartoma of hair follicle tissue typically occurring on the face of adults. Trichofolliculoma are pilosebaceous in origin.

16. D) Causes of erythema nodosum include birth control pills, oestrogens, cat-scratch disease, fungal diseases, infectious mononucleosis, sarcoidosis, Behcet's disease, inflammatory bowel diseases, tuberculosis, streptococcal infection, mycoplasma pneumoniae, Epstein-Barr virus, medications (sulfonamides), pregnancy and cancer.

17. B) The Scl-antibody, also known as antitoposomerase antibody is a blood test that is most commonly associated with systemic sclerosis, also known as scleroderma. Scl-70 is present approximately 60% time in the limited variant of systemic sclerosis.

18. A) In persons with drug-induced lupus erythe-mátosus, anti-Sm antibodies are rare. An anti-histone antibody that is often implicated in drug- induced lupus erythematosus is immunoglobulin G (anti-[H2A-H2B] DNA). Anti-histone antibodies are much more likely to indicate drug-induced lupus erythematosus; however can also appear as many as 50% of patients with SLE. Anti-nuclear antibody yields positive results in many connective tissue disorders and other autoimmune diseases, and may occur in normal individuals. Subtypes of anti-Smith and double stranded DNA (ds DNA) antibodies are linked to SLE and antihistone antibodies are linked to drug lupus.

19. A) Erythroderma may cause thickening and flaking of skin. Peeling of skin occurs in exfoliative dermatitis, eczema, psoriasis, and ichthyosis, Kawasaki disease, a disorder usually found among infant and young children causes rash and swelling of the hands. Scarlet fever sometimes causes rashes over the upper body, which spreads throughout the entire body.

20. D) The most common cause of chronic leg ulcers is poor blood circulation in the legs. These are known as arterial and venous leg ulcers.

Causes of leg ulcers include trauma, systemic sclerosis, diabetes, vascular disease, (stroke, angina, heart attack,) tumours and infection. They may also caused especially impetigo, ecthyma, cellulitis, and less often in tuberculosis and leprosy. They are common in all haemolytic anaemias. In sickle cell anaemia large indolent and deep ulcers are formed most commonly around ankle of the older child. Stasis of RBCs has a major role.

21. C) Brooke's tumour or trichoepithelioma derived from the hair follicle appearing as a firm flesh coloured nodule, usually on the face. The non-hereditary tumour is generally seen in early adult life.

22. D) Tinea barbae or barbae itch is involvement of the bearded areas of face and neck. Tinea pedis is most often due to infection by trichophyton rubrum. Onychomycosis is fungal infection of nail.

23. D) Carbuncle is caused by staphylococcus. Staphylococcus, and beta haemolytic streptococci cause impetigo. Erysipelas is caused by group A streptococci. Taenia capitis or alopecia that may progress to severely inflamed deep abscesses termed kerion, with the potential for scarring and permanent alopacia.

24. C) Skin appendages include sweat glands, apocrine sweat glands and sebaceous glands.

25. C) Common warts are termed verruca vulgaris. They appear as hyperkeratotic papules with a rough, irregular surface. They range from smaller than 1 mm to larger than 1 cm. They can occur on any part of the body but are seen more commonly on the hands and knees. Flat warts also termed plane warts or verruca plana. Deep palmoplantar warts are termed myrmecia. Genital wart (or condyloma accuminata and anogenital warts) is a highly contagious sexually transmitted disease caused by human papilloma virus.

26. B) Seborrhoeic keratoses are very common harmless skin lesions that appear during adult life. Seborrhoeic keratoses may also be called basal cell papillomas, senile warts or brown warts. They begin as slightly raised, skin coloured or light brown spots. Gradually they thicken and take on a rough, warty surface. They slowly darken and may turn black.

27. B) The lesions are usually multiple, each consisting of a discrete waxy skin coloured papule which may grow to about 5 mm in diameter with a central depression from which paste like material can be expressed.

28. A) Corps ronds are pathognomic of Darier's disease. Dyskeratotic round cells occurring in the epidermis with a central round basophilic mass surrounded by a clear halo, characteristically found in Darier's disease. Corps ronds are predominantly located in stratum spinosum and stratum granulosum.

29. C) There are two types of dermatitis

a. Irritant contact dermatitis

b. Allergic contact dermatitis.

Patch testing can help to differentiate between two. The test involves the application of various test substances to the skin under adhesive tape that left in place for 48 hours. The skin is then examined a further 48 hours later for any response. Allergic dermatitis due to specific allergen test is positive. Weak positive reactions are slightly elevated pink or red plaques.

Strong positives are papulovesicles and extreme reactions are blisters or ulcers.

30. A) von-Recklinghausen's neurofibromatosis is also called von-Recklinghausen disease or simply neurofibromatosis. It is an autosomal dominant hereditary disorder caused by a single gene. Patients develop multiple soft tissue tumours (neurofibromas) and very often skin spots (freckling and café-au-lait). The tumour occurs under the skin and through out the nervous system.

31. C) The etiology of psoriasis is unknown. Infections by various microorganisms, metabolic disturbances, endocrine dysfunction, neurogenic factors, and trauma, as well as parturition have been considered important precipitating factors.

32. A) Nodular basal cell carcinoma is the most common type of basal cell carcinoma and present as round, pearly flesh coloured papule with telangiectases. As it enlarges, it frequently ulcerates centrally leaving a raised, pearly border with telangiectases, which aids in making a diagnosis.

33. B) Staphylococcal Scalded Skin Syndrome has also been called Ritter's disease or Lyell's disease. It is an illness characterized by red blistering skin that looks like a burn or scalds hence its name staphylococcal scalded skin syndrome. SSSS is caused by release of epidermolytic toxins A and B from toxigenic strains of the bacteria staphylococcus aureus.

34. C) Civette bodies (colloid bodies) are found in lichen planus. Civette bodies are eosinophilic hyaline spherical bodies seen in or just beneath the epidermis particularly in lichen planus. They are formed by necrosis of individual basal cells.

35. B) In lichen planus rete ridges of epidermis are long and pointed, like the teeth of a saw. Other histological features of lichen planus are hyperkeratosis of epidermis, liquefaction degeneration of basal layer, and dense infiltration of lymphocytes along the dermoepidermal junction.

36. D) White sponge nevus.

Cannon described it in 1935.

It is also known as Cannon's disease or hereditary leukokeratosis of mucosa, appears to follow hereditary pattern as an autosomal dominant trait.

Cause: It is caused by mutation of keratin 4 and keratin 13 genes.

Clinical features:

White sponge nevus almost always presents during childhood and there is no gender predilection.

It presents in the mouth, most frequently as a thick bilateral white plaque with a spongy texture, usually on the buccal mucosa, but sometimes on the labial mucosa, alveolar ridge, or floor of the mouth. The gingival margin and dorsum of the tongue are almost never affected.

Individual lesions are seen as a relatively thick, white, often corrugated plaque, which may cover most of the oral mucosa. Usually asymptomatic, rare examples of mild discomfort have been reported from secondary infection.

Microscopically: There is marked intercellular edema of the superficial epithelial cells, predominantly within the spinous layer. The nuclei are typically pyknotic and the cells may mimic the koilocytes of viral infection. Edematous cells may be organized into inverted triangles with broad bases along the surface, and there may be a thickened parakeratin layer.

37. C) The malignant transformation of oral erosive and atrophic lesions has been described 0.3 percent to 12.5 percent. The development of squamous cell carcinoma may occur in areas directly affected by lichen planus, as well as other areas of the oral mucosa. However, it is not established if atrophic and erosive forms of lichen planus have an intrinsic potential for malignant transformation or if the disorder facilitates the development of oral mucosa squamous cell carcinoma of exogenous carcinogen.

38. C) In cases of erythema multiformae patient presents with a polymorphic eruption of erythematous macules, blisters, urticarial plaques, vesicles, bullae, erosions and target lesions (concentric, circular erythematous rings resembling a target or bulls eye). Target lesions are dusky round; maculopapules appear suddenly in a symmetric pattern on the backs of hands and feet and the extensor aspect of forearms and legs.

39. C) Bullous lesions of skin

Solar/thermal injury
Bullous impetigo
Herpes simplex
Varicella infection
Pemphigus
Pemphigoid
Erythema multiformae
Porphyria
SLE
Epidermolysis bullosa
Dermatitis herpetiformis
Staphylococcal scalded skin syndrome
Graft versus host disease
Drug reaction

40. B) Café-au-lait spots are pigmented birthmarks.

Causes of Café-au-lait spots are:

Neurofibromatosis
McCune-Albright syndrome
Legius syndrome
Tuberous sclerosis
Fanconi anaemia
Idiopathic
Ataxia telangiectasia
Bloom syndrome
Chediak-Higashi syndrome
Gaucher's disease
Hunter syndrome
Wiskott-Aldrich syndrome
Maffucci syndrome
Multiple mucosal neuroma syndrome

41. A) Junctional nevus is characterized by nests of nevus cells along the basal layer of the epithelium. The nevi cells are cuboidal, oval, or spindle shaped. Cytoplasm is distinctly outlined. Nuclei are large round or oval. Some of these cells drop off into underlying connective tissue, showing junctional activity.

42. B) In cases of erythema multiformae patient presents with a polymorphic eruption of erythematous macules, blisters, urticarial plaques, vesicles, bullae, erosions and target lesions (concentric, circular erythematous rings resembling a target or bulls eye). Target lesions are dusky round; maculopapules appear suddenly in a symmetric pattern on the backs of hands and feet and the extensor aspect of forearms and legs.

43. D) The cutaneous lesions of congenital syphilis are very characteristics. Within the first seven days of birth, a bullous eruption may develop.

It consists of bullae distributed bilaterally and symmetrically on the front of the wrists, palms, ankles, and soles, later bullae develops on the other parts of the body.

44. C) In borderline tuberculoid leprosy the resistance to the M. leprae is somewhat less than tuberculoid patients and the clinical aspect of the lesion reflects this. Satellite lesions indicate local spread of the disease occurring due to a decrease in the patient's defense mechanism (cell mediated immunity) and are characteristic of borderline tuberculoid leprosy. The characteristic lesions in borderline tuberculoid leprosy are hyperpigmented, anaesthetic small, and satellite.

45. C) Borderline lepromatous leprosy lesions may be erythematous or copper coloured infiltrated patches, raised in the centre (dome-shaped) and sloping towards the periphery, presenting an inverted saucer appearance.

46. D) Children with kwashiorkor have characteristic skin lesions, with alternating zones of hyperpigmentation, areas of desquamation, and hypopigmentation, giving a "flaky, paint appearance".

47. A) Lichen planus is a chronic autoimmune inflammatory condition affecting the lining of the mouth. The exact cause is unknown but an immune pathogenesis is suspected, as there is an association with some autoimmune diseases such as myasthenia gravis, thymoma, alopecia, areata, dermatomyositis, primary biliary cirrhosis, ulcerative colitis, and graft versus host reaction. Oral lichen planus is a T mediated autoimmune disease in which cytotoxic CD8+T cells trigger the apoptosis of oral epithelial cells. The lesional CD8+T cells being more cytotoxic—may produce lymphokines, interferon, and tumour necrosis factor.

48. B) Gottron papule is erythematous, and atrophic papules are found over the knuckles and pressure points characteristically seen in dermatomyositis.

49. B) Bullous pemphigoid is an uncommon subepidermal blistering disease typically presenting on the flexor surface of elderly patients. Begins with a localized area of erythema or with pruritic urticarial plaques. Plaques turn dark red in 1 to 3 weeks as vesicles and bullae rapidly appear on their surfaces.

Microscopically: Subepidermal bullae in dermis and bullae cavity show lymphocytes or eosinophilic infiltration. These cells are chiefly perivascular and are predominantly eosinophils. In severe inflammation, the basal keratocytes of mesenchymal demonstrates spongiosis. There is basal layer vacuolation. The vacuolated basal layer eventually gives rise to a fluid-filled blister.

Pathogenesis

There is linear deposition of immunoglobulin IgG autoantibodies and complement in the basement membrane zone.

IgG autoantibodies bind to the skin basement membrane of patients with bullous pemphigoid.

The antigen concerned in these lesions is named as *"Bullous pemphigoid antigen" (BP230 BpAg1) and BP180 (BPAg2)*. It is present at dermoepidermal junction.

Direct immunofluorescence shows immunoglobulin G (IgG), complement C3 or both in a linear band at the basement membrane zone.

50. B) Pemphigoid

Microscopically: Subepidermal bullae in dermis and bullae cavity show lymphocytes or eosinophilic infiltration. These cells are chiefly perivascular and are predominantly eosinophils. In severe inflammation, the basal keratocytes of mesenchymal demonstrates spongiosis. There is basal layer vacuolation. The vacuolated basal layer eventually gives rise to a fluid-filled blister.

Pemphigus

Microscopically shows intraepithelial bullae, acantholysis, and a mild to moderate infiltrate of eosinophils. The basal keratocytes, although separated from one another through the loss of attachment, remain firmly attached to the dermis like a *"row of tomb stones"*.

Stevens Johnson's syndrome

Microscopically

Early stage: Vacuolization of basal keratocytes and individual cell necrosis throughout the epidermis.

Late stage: Full thickness epidermal necrosis and detachment with formation of subepidermal split above basement membrane. There is little or no inflammatory infiltrate in dermis.

Psoriasis

Histological findings demonstrates:

1. Confluent parakeratosis.
2. Acanthosis with regular elongation of the rete ridges with thickening in their lower portion.
3. Thinning of the suprapapillary epidermis with the occasional presence of small spongiform pustules.
4. Munro microabscess of neutrophils superficially.
5. Pallor of the upper layer of epidermis.
6. Diminished to absent granular layer.
7. Elongation and edema of dermal papillae.
8. Chronic inflammation of sub-epidermal layer with polymorphonuclear leukocytes, lymphocytes, and histocytes.
9. Dilated and tortuous blood vessels high in the submucosa.

51. B) Actinic keratosis (also called "solar keratosis) is a premalignant condition of thick, scaly or crusty patches of skin. It progresses to squamous cell carcinoma. Squamous cell carcinoma can be a complication of chronic ulcers.

Lupus vulgaris (known as tuberculosis luposa) is painful cutaneous tuberculosis. Skin lesions with nodular appearances, most often on the face, around nose, eyelids, cheeks, and ears.

Marjolin's ulcer refers to an aggressive squamous cell carcinoma presenting in an area of previously traumatized, chronically inflamed or scarred skin. They are commonly present in the context of chronic wounds including burn injuries, venous ulcers, ulcers from osteomyelitis.

52. A) Pyoderma gangrenosum is thought to be due to immune system dysfunction and particularly improper functioning of neutrophils.

Skin reactions in internal malignancy:

1. Some inflammatory reactions occurring in the skin may also signal internal malignancy e.g., pruritis, a very common problem.
2. Metastases to the skin occur in up to five percent of patients who have internal malignancy.
3. A cellulitis type of inflammatory response is occasionally seen e.g., Paget's disease of nipple.
4. Purpura may be the earliest sign in leukaemia especially the granulocytic and monocytic types.
5. Migratory phlebitis is an uncommon but fairly characteristic sign of internal malignancy.
6. Erythema nodosum may be found reasonably often in patients with malignancy or lymphoma.
7. Erythema multiformae is most common of the vesiculobullous eruption.
8. Other bullous lesions are bullous pemphigoid and herpetiformis.
9. Urticaria is by far the commonest of the reactive erythemas.
10. Erythema annulare centrifugan is an annular or arciform pattern erythematous reaction of the skin.

11. Exfoliative erythroderma is uncommon, and may be due to an extensive dermatosis such as psoriasis, lichen planus or seborrheic dermatitis. When malignancy is cause it is most likely to be a lymphoma or leukaemia.
12. Diffuse pigmentation of the skin has been reported in extensive malignant melanoma and pituitary tumours.
13. An addisonian type of pigmentation may be seen if the adrenals are involved by carcinoma or leukaemia.

53. B) Granuloma inguinale (donovanosis) does affect regional lymph nodes, but this is rare.

In cases of syphilis the trepenomes spread through lymphatic vessels to the regional lymph nodes where they multiply. About one week after development of primary chancre, the inguinal lymph nodes begin to enlarge. They are painless and can be palpated bilaterally, and have a rubbery consistency. If the chancre is situated at the cervix, inguinal lymph node enlargement is usually not present because of lymphatic drainage to the deep pelvic lymph nodes.

Chancroid: Haemophilus Ducreyi is the sexually transmitted micro-organism responsible for chancroid.

Two to twenty days later, half of the cases show a painful lymph node enlargement in one or sometimes both inguinal areas. The nodes can become confluent, forming an oval fluctuating uniocular abscess (bubo), which is covered by a reddish skin. The bubo can break, by first forming a sinus which is followed by a large ulcer.

Lymphogranuloma venereum is caused by chlamydia trachomatis. There is involvement of inguinal lymph node swelling about two weeks after infection.

54. A) 1. **Superficial spreading melanoma**

Superficial-spreading melanoma is the most common subtype, accounting for 70 to 80% of all melanomas arising in a preexisting lesion. They are common on the trunk in men and on the legs in women. The lesion tends to be larger than 6 mm in diameter, flat, asymmetric with varying colouration. Invasive malignant melanoma generally develops from superficial melanoma in situ in 5 to 10 years.

Microscopically it is characterized by presence of buckshot (pagetoid) scatter of atypical melanocytes within the epidermis.

Hutchinson's freckle: Lentigo maligna melanoma represents 5% to 10% of all cases of melanoma. It occurs on the damaged skin of face in elderly people. It arises from a brown macular lesion called lentigo maligna or Hutchinson's freckle. The lesion is brown with some variation in epidermal pigment density. It has got predilection for exposed parts. As the disease advances, invasion and metastasis are frequent.

55. A) Lepromin test indicates host resistance to M. Leprae. It does not confirm the diagnosis but useful in determining the type of leprosy. A positive test is indicative of cell-mediated immunity, which is seen in tuberculoid leprosy. A negative test suggests a lack of resistance to disease and is seen in lepromatous leprosy. A negative test indicates a poorer prognosis.

To do this test, bacillary suspension is injected into the forearm. When the reaction is read at 48 hours it is called the Fernandez reaction and indicates delayed hypersensitivity to antigens of M. leprae or mycobacterium that cross react. When it is read at 3-4 weeks it is called the Mitsuda reaction and indicates the person is capable of mounting an efficient response.

56. C) In cases of Madura foot the fungal grain discharge from sinuses is thin and serous and contains the diagnostic "golden yellow" granules called **sulphur granules.** The material discharged from the sinuses is in the form of grains consisting of colonies of fungi or bacteria. They are 1 to 3 mm in diameter but may coalesce and form larger aggregations, several millimeters in diameter.

Histologically: The granule is found to contain entangled mycelia in the center embedded in pus, forming minute abscesses with a large number of monocytes, polymorphs and plasma cells. The diagnostic feature is the presence of granules.

57. A) Wood's lamp is a mercury vapor ultraviolet lamp with a filter of barium silicate glass with 9% nickel oxide. The filter allows UV light in the wavelength of 320 to 400 nanometers only while blocking out all. Other wavelengths. Wood's lamp mainly emits ultraviolet light in the wavelength of 360 nanometers.

Wood's lamp examination is to detect several conditions affecting skin, including:

1. Bacterial infections
2. Fungal infections—Taenia capitis
3. Porphyria
4. Skin colouring changes
5. Tuberous sclerosis (Epiloia)

Taenia capitis, the fungal infection of scalp, is caused by different species of fungi. Examination of scalp in darkroom with Wood's lamp produces a greenish fluorescence when the infection is caused by certain species like microsporum and trichophyton schoenleini.

Wood's lamp fluoresce a coral pink colour in erythresma, a superficial bacterial infection causing brownish red patches on the skin. A yellowish green fluorescence is typical of pseudomonas infection.

In dark coloured skinned individuals it may be difficult to distinguish between normal skin and slightly hypopigmented areas in diseases like pityriasis versicolour, pityriasis alba and leaf macules present in tuberous sclerosis (epiloia).

Melasma and freckles, the level of melanin deposition can be differentiated using Wood's lamp.

Dark colour due to pigments in the outer epidermal layer of skin is accentuated while the colour of upper dermal pigments is decreased during Wood's lamp examination.

Examination of urine with a Wood's lamp: may reveal coral pink fluorescence due to excessive porphyrins.

58. D. Premalignant lesions of skin include

1. Solar keratosis
2. Radiation dermatosis
3. Bowen's disease
4. Proliferative verrucous leukoplakia
5. Lichen planus

59. C) Cock peculiar tumour is a sebaceous cyst linked growth. Chronic inflammation causes the cyst to take the form of granuloma. The most common sites are scalp and scrotum.

60. A) Marjolin's ulcer refers to an aggressive squamous cell carcinoma presenting in an area of previously traumatized, chronically inflamed or scarred skin. They are commonly present in the context of chronic wounds including burn injuries, venous ulcers, ulcers from osteomyelitis.

Tuberculous ulcer is known as lupus vulgaris.

Basal cell carcinoma is called rodent ulcer.

61. B) Basal cell carcinomas never metastasize therefore always primary lesion. Basal cell carcinomas arise in the basal cells of the pilosebaceous adnexa and occur only on the skin. Mucosal surfaces lacking these adnexa such as cervix, lips, and tongue are never primary sites.

62. C) In cases of cryptococcus neoformans diagnosis is by isolation of organisms in sputum, cerebrospinal fluid, pus and brain tissue by smear and culture.

In maduramycosis diagnosis is by demonstration of organisms in sulphur granules from discharging sinus (skin).

In blastomycosis, skin lesions are usually asymptomatic, appear as ulcerated lesions with small pustules at the margins. Fungus can be demonstrated in skin smear.

Tinia versicolor: Pityriasis versicolor is a mild, chronic superficial fungal infection of the stratum corneum characterized by white brown or fawn coloured discrete to confluent lesions covered with thin scales. It is caused by malassezia furfur, affects the upper chest, back, abdomen, neck and upper arms, and shows macules with peripheral scaling.

Fungus can be demonstrated in skin smear.

chapter 17

OPHTHALMIC PATHOLOGY

1. Snow ball opacity in vitreous is seen in?
   A) Pars planitis
   B) Sarcoidosis
   C) Toxoplasmosis
   D) Fuch's lesion
2. Ocular manifestations of neurofibromatosis include:
   A) Plexiform tumour of lids with ptosis
   B) Glioma of optic nerves
   C) Congenital glaucoma
   D) All of the above
3. The following factors are important in angiogenesis in diabetic retinopathy except:
   A) Tissue necrosis factor
   B) Basic fibroblast growth factor
   C) Insulin like growth factor
   D) Vascular endothelial growth factor
4. Optic atrophy occur in deficiency of following vitamin B:
   A) Vitamin B_2
   B) Vitamin B_3
   C) Vitamin B_6
   D) Vitamin B_{12}
5. Microaneurysms are except:
   A) Are dilatation of retinal vein
   B) Can be distinguished from dot haemorrhage by fluorescein angiography
   C) Are 10 μm to 100 μm in diameter
   D) Are usually found in areas of retinal Non-perfusion
6. Characteristic eye sign in dysthyroid states is:
   A) Exophthalamos
   B) Ptosis
   C) Optic neuroatrophy
   D) Myopathy
7. Flexner-Wintersteiner rosettes occur in:
   A) Retinoblastoma
   B) Neuroblastoma
   C) Medulloblastoma
   D) Choroidal melanoma
8. Choose the correct answer the following corneal conditions are autosomal recessive
   A) Granular dystrophy
   B) Macular dystrophy
   C) Lattice dystrophy
   D) Meesman's dystrophy
9. Most common second malignancy in survivors of retinoblstoma is:
   A) Thyroid carcinoma
   B) Nasopharyngeal carcinoma
   C) Optic glioma
   D) Osteosarcoma
10. Cherry red spots in all except:
    A) Niemann Pick disease
    B) Multiple sulphatase deficiency
    C) Krabbe disease
    D) Type II glycoprotein
11. "Cotton wool" spot's in the retina are indicative of?
    A) Microaneurysm

B) Microinfarcts
C) Proteinaceous material
D) None of the above

12. The commonest conjunctival tumour is:
A) Basal cell carcinoma
B) Adenoid cystic carcinoma
C) Squamous cell carcinoma
D) Malignant melanoma

13. Which of the following HLA is not associated with an increased incidence of uveitis?
A) HLA B27
B) HLA-A29
C) HLA-B51
D) HLA –A1

14. All of the following are responsible for blindness in children except:
A) Dacrocystitis
B) Glaucoma
C) Malnutrition
D) Ophthalmia neonatorum

15. Cat eye syndrome is associated with:
A) Partial trisomy 21
B) Partial trisomy 18.
C) Partial trisomy 13
D) Partial trisomy 22

16. The following are prognostic importance in choroidal melanoma except:
A) Size of tumour
B) Location of tumour
C) Presence of blood vessels within tumour cells
D) Type of tumour cells

17. Most common lymphoma of orbit is:
A) Hodgkin's lymphoma
B) Diffuse Large B-cell type
C) Follicular type
D) MALT lymphoma

18. Ocular features of trisomy 13 include except:
A) Optic nerve hypoplasia
B) Microphthalmia
C) Iris coloboma
D) Corneal opacities

19. Halbersteadter-Prowazeke's bodies are seen in:
A) Yellow fever
B) Leishmaniasis
C) Trachoma
D) Lymphogranuloma venereum

20. Cause of ophthalmia neonatorum is:
A) Gonorrhoea
B) Syphilis
C) Human papilloma virus infection
D) AIDS

21. Most common ophthalmic lesion in toxoplasmosis is:
A) Chorioretinitis
B) Hard exudates
C) Conjunctivitis
D) Corneal sclerosis

22. Bare orbit is seen in all/except
A) Neurofibromatosis
B) Metastasis
C) Haemangioma
D) Meningioma

23. Orbital metastasis commonly occurs from al /except:
A) Bronchus
B) Kidney
C) Gastrointestinal tract
D) Ovaries

Answers

1. B) Snow ball or string pearl type of vitreou opacities is known as a sign of sarcoidc sis. The opacities are mostly situated in th inferior vitreous.

2. D) Neurofibromatosis type-1 (NF-1)–morbu von-Recklinghausen disease is an autosc mal dominant phacomatosis. The gene NI 1 is located on chromosome 17.11.2. Ocu lar manifestation of neurofibromatosis NI 1 include plexiform neurofibroma of eye lid with ptosis, uveal melanocytic nev Lisch nodules in 97% of cases, retina glioma, hamartomas, congenital glau coma, optic nerve glioma, pulsating exophthalamos (due to absence of the sphenoidal ring).

3. A) Vascular endothelial growth factor is a chemical signal produced by cells that stimulates the growth of new blood vessels. VEGF is also important in diabetic retinopathy. Many authors also consider insulin like growth factor-1 and basic fibroblast growth factor the angiogenic agent.

4. D) Optic atrophy occurs in vitamin B_{12} deficiency

5. A) Increasing numbers of microaneurysms are associated with capillary occlusion, visible on fluoresin angiography leading to retinal ischemia (lack of oxygen) and progression of retinopathy. They are small round dark red dots on the retinal surface. This tiny aneurysm varies from 20 to 100 microns in diameter and situated in areas of non-perfusion.

6. A) Commonest eye sign in dysthyroid state is exophthalamos. Exophthalamos is a condition of altered thyroid metabolism that causes protein depositions within the extraocular muscles. The etiology of the thyroid-related orbitopathy is an autoimmune mediated inflammatory process of the orbital tissue predominantly affecting fat and extraocular muscles.

7. A) Retinoblastoma is the most common intraocular malignancy in children. A feature of retinoblastoma includes the formation of Flexner-Winterstein rosettes, which are formation of retinal differentiation. The cells of these rosettes surround a central lumen.

8. B) Macular dystrophy is inherited by the autosomal recessive method, which means that it may be more severe than other types of dystrophy. It may appear before the age of 20 years. Granular dystrophy, lattice dystrophy, and Meesman's dystrophy are inherited by the dominant method.

9. D) Most common second malignancy in survivors of retinoblastoma is osteogenic sarcoma.

10. C) A cherry red spot is a finding in the macula in a variety of lipid storage disorders. It describes the appearance of a small circular choroid shape, as seen through fovea centralis. Cherry red spots are seen in central retinal artery occlusion, Tay-Sach's disease, Niemann-Pick disease, Sandhoff's disease, Gaucher's disease, sialodosis, gangliosidosis, metachromatic leukodystrophy and multiple sulphatase deficiency.

11. B) Cotton wool spots are small areas of yellowish white colouration in the retina, which consists of nerve fibres. This swelling almost always occurs because the blood supply to that areas has been impaired and in the absence of normal blood flow through the retinal vessels the nerve fibres are injured in a particular location resulting in swelling and the appearance of a cotton wool spot. The most common causes of a cotton wool spots are diseases, which affect the retina, such as diabetes, and high blood pressure.

12. C) Most common conjunctival cancer is squamous cell carcinoma. Other malignant tumours arises from conjunctiva include malignant melanoma and lymphoma.

13. D) Acute anterior uveitis is associated with rheumatic disorders such as ankylosing spondylitis. HLA-27 antigen is present in 98% of these cases. HLA-A29 is the strongest association of a specific HLA with human disease syndrome, birdshot retinochoroidopathy. HLA-B51 is strongly associated with Behcet's disease.

14. A) Causes of blindness in children include anophathamos, microphthalmos, corneal scarring, keratoconus, cataract, aphakia, aniridia, retinal dystrophy, glaucoma, vitamin A deficiency disorders, trauma, ophthalmia neonatorum, and neonatal conjunctivtis.

15. D) Cat eye syndrome named after how it affects the appearance of the eyes, is caused by a genetic defect in chromosome 22. Wide range of symptoms is associated with the syndrome. They are iris coloboma, small growths of skin (tag), or depressions in the skin (pits) of the outer ears and an absence or anus (anal atresia), congenital heart defects and cleft palate.

16. C) Several clinical and pathological prognostic factors have been identified that are associated with higher risk of metastasis of uveal melanomas. These include large tumour size, ciliary body involvement, location of tumors, presence of orange pigment overlying the tumour, and older patient.

Site of tumour: An anteriorly situated tumour has poor prognosis.

Tumour size: Larger tumour has poorer prognosis.

Cell type: Epitheloid cells have poor prognosis than spindle cell type.

Age of patient: Older patients have poor prognosis.

Other features associated with an increase risk of mortality include optic nerve extension, size of retinal detachment and extrascleral spread.

17. B) According to REAL, the commonest subtypes of lymphoma originating in orbit are the extranodal diffuse large B-cell lymphoma. MALT lymphoma can arise from lacrimal gland, which is conjunctival origin. The remainder low grade lymphoma of the orbit are those types most commonly encountered as orbital primaries are follicular lymphoma, small cell B-lymphocytic lymphoma, rarely mantle cell lymphoma.

18. D) Ocular features of trisomy 13 include:

1. Retinal detachment
2. Retinal dysplasia
3. Cataract
4. Nystagmus
5. Cortical visual loss
6. Optic nerve hypoplasia
7. Microphthalmia
8. Persistent hyperplastic primary vitreous

19. C) Halberstaedter-Prowazeke's bodies are seen in trachoma.

Halberstaedter-Powazeke's bodies (trachoma bodies) are distinctive complex, intracytoplasmic forms found in the conjunctival epithelial cells of persons in the acute phase of trachoma, less frequently in later stages varying from:

1. Discrete acidophilic granules (approximately 250 nm in diameter).
2. Irregular clumps of such material embedded in basophilic matrix.
3. Relatively large basophilic body's (approximately 700-1000 nm in diameter).
4. Large basophilic body's that include discrete tiny acidophilic granules.

20. A) Ophthalmia neonatorum is a severe acute conjunctivitis with a copious purulent discharge especially in newborn, caused by Neisseria gonorrhoeae. Neisseria gonorrhoeae manifest earliest, typically within the first 48 hours of birth.

The conjunctiva becomes intensely inflamed, bright red and swollen, with a thick yellow pus discharge.

Complications include corneal ulcer and opacity, prolapsed iris, adherent leucoma, panophthalmitis, metastatic stomatitis and arthritis.

21. A) The most common finding in congenital toxoplasmosis is the ophthalmic manifestation retinochoroiditis, which has a predilection for the posterior lobe.

Toxoplasmosis causes a necrotizing retiniti, often there will be an old scar with an area of reactivation at the edge of the scar. This is seen as a focal retinitis, vitreous cells and vasculitis.

22. C) Causes of bare orbit

1. Neurofibromatosis
2. Meningioma
3. Optic glioma
4. Aneurysm
5. Retinoblastoma
6. Idiopathic
7. Eosinophilic granuloma
8. Metastasis

Bare orbit: The characteristic anomaly of unilateral dysplasia of the wings of the sphenoid is called bare orbit.

Bare orbit appearance is seen in neurofibromatosis due to sphenoid dysplasia, metastasis due to destruction and meningioma due to sclerosis.

23. D) Orbital metastasis is relatively uncommon, but some primary tumours do have a predilection to metastasize to the orbit.

Common tumours to metastasize the orbit Include:

A) Breast tumour

B) Bronchogenic carcinoma

C) Prostate cancer

D) Gastrointestinal adenocarcinoma

E) Thyroid carcinoma

F) Renal cell carcinoma

G) Neuroblastoma

H) Ewing's sarcoma

I) Wilm's tumour.

Some exciting gifts are up for grabs with this book!!

MCQ PATHOLOGY

Dr Mrinalini Sant

FREE Gifts Rs. 1000/-

DEAR READERS

By now you must have gone through this book in the entirety. So we invite your assessment on this title with absolute impartiality and candid observations. After all, we publishers blindly depend on your benchmarking. Friends, please fill up the open spaces below with CAPITAL LETTERS. You may add some extra sheets of paper if the space provided is not sufficient for you.

i. What are the important topics of your syllabus which are not adequately covered in this book?

ii. In which chapters and on what topics the treatment of the subject-matter by the author is not satisfactory and why?

iii. Have you come across the typos, factual inaccuracies, inconsistencies, and other forms of mistakes in the book? If yes, then please specify the mistakes and page numbers.

iv. Name top three books on the same subject, which, in your consideration, are better than this book. Could you provide some reasons?

Your 1st Preference: ....

Your 2nd Preference: ....

Your 3rd Preference: ....

v. Any suggestion to improve the quality of illustrations, diagrams, etc.?

vi. How did you like the cover design? Any suggestion on colours?

vii. Suggestions for further improvement of production-standard:

viii. Who recommended you this book:

☐ Teacher ☐ Friend ☐ Parents ☐ Bookseller ☐ Librarian

ix. Name of the person who has recommended:

Designation: ....

Address: ....

Phone No.: ....

e-mail: ....

x. Name and address of the bookseller from whom you have purchased this book:

....

....

....

xi. Name and address of the library where you would like to find the book:

....

....

xii. Name and address of your institution (Please mention the University or Board):

....

....

xiii. Your name, e-mail, and complete postal address:

....

....

....

xiv. A few other titles published by us that you would like to read:

....

....

The best assessment will be rewarded half-yearly. The award will be in the form of our publications, as decided by the Editorial and Marketing Operations Division, amounting to Rs. 1000/- (Rupees one thousand) only.

....

Please mail the filled up coupon at your earliest to :

Editorial & Marketing Operations Division

NEW CENTRAL BOOK AGENCY (P) Ltd

8/1 Chintamoni Das Lane, Kolkata 700 009

West Bengal, INDIA

Phone + Fax: 033 + 2241 8411, 2241 8573, 2241 9094

e-mail: ncbapvtltd@eth.net, ncba@cal2.vsnl.net.in

Website: www.centralgroup.com